CHILDHOOD INCONTINENCE

A guide to problems of wetting and soiling for parents and professionals

CHILDHOOD INCONTINENCE

A guide to problems of wetting
and soiling for parents and
professionals

ROGER MORGAN BA (Wales), PhD (Leicester)

Illustrations by Bill Brennan

Published for the
DISABLED LIVING FOUNDATION

by
HEINEMANN MEDICAL BOOKS LTD.
London

First published 1981

©The Disabled Living Foundation 1981
346 Kensington High Street
London W.14.

ISBN 0 433 22220 4

Phototypeset by G. Over Limited, Rugby and Harrow and printed by Redwood Burn Ltd., Trowbridge, Wilts.

CONTENTS

	page
Preface	ix
Acknowledgements	x
Forewords	xi

1 Introduction — 1

2 Bladder and bowel control — what do they mean? — 4
   The structure and working of the bladder — 4
   The structure and working of the bowel — 7
   The basic skills: — 9
     1 Postponing urination — 9
     2 Keeping the rectum empty — 10
     3 Perceiving the need to empty — 11
     4 Starting the urine stream — 11
     5 Starting defaecation — 12
     6 Monitoring and responding while asleep — 12
     7 Knowing when and where to 'go' — 14
     8 Coping with clothing, cleaning and toilet equipment — 14
   Learning the skills — taught or just acquired? — 14
   Toilet training and its effects — 16
     1 Daytime 'potting' — 16
     2 Night-time 'potting' — 17
     3 Encouragement and praise — 18
     4 Punishment — 18
     5 Changes in circumstances — 18
     6 Restricting fluids — 18
     7 Demonstration — 19
   Conclusion — encouraging continence — 20

3 The problem of bedwetting — 21
   Nature and frequency — 21
     Deliberate wetting — 21
     How many children wet the bed? — 22
     Sex ratio — 22
     Social class — 22

	The beginning of the problem	22
	Bedwetting in families	23
	The origins of bedwetting	24
	Emotional stress	24
	Individual differences	24
	Infection	25
	Abnormalities	25
	Deep sleep	26
	Emotional disturbance	26
	Common ways of helping the bedwetting child	26
	Lifting	27
	Punishment	27
	Rewards	28
	Star charts	28
	Restricting fluids	28
	Common forms of treatment	29
	Reassurance	30
	Drug treatments	30
	Psychotherapy	31
	The enuresis alarm or 'buzzer'	31
4	**How 'buzzer' treatment works**	**33**
	The basic idea	33
	The ways in which control is learned	35
	Effectiveness	38
	Can success or failure be predicted?	39
5	**Using the enuresis alarm ('buzzer') at home**	**41**
	Suitability of the treatment	41
	Medical contact	41
	Types of apparatus	42
	Setting up the progress record	46
	Practical considerations before treatment	50
	Stresses	50
	Previous experience of treatment	51
	Sleeping arrangements	51
	Bedding	51
	More than one bedwetter	52
	Explaining to the child	52
	Setting up the apparatus	53

Nightly routine	56
Signs of progress	58
More urine to 'finish off' in the toilet	58
Smaller wet patches	59
Only one wet per night	59
Better waking to the alarm	59
Reduced daytime problems	59
More dry nights	59
Self-waking to visit the toilet	60
The end of treatment and overlearning	60
Relapse after treatment	61
Problems and solutions	61
Not waking to the alarm	62
Not 'shutting off' the stream of urine	63
Damaged or worn detector mats	64
False alarms	64
Alarm failure	65
Alarm treatment with the handicapped child	65

6 Daytime pants wetting — 68

Nature and incidence	68
Urgency and frequency	68
Stress incontinence	69
'Giggle micturition'	69
Ways of improving the situation	70
Holding practice	70
Controlling urgency	72
Pelvic floor exercises	74
Coping with smell	75
Formal treatments	75
Treatment of infection	75
Medicines	75
Daytime enuresis alarm or 'buzzer'	76
Teaching daytime control to the mentally handicapped	77
Analysing the problem	78
Planning and using a training programme	78

7 Soiling — 83

Types of soiling	83
Retention-with-overflow	83

Non-control	85
Staining	86
Countermeasures to soiling	86
Regular toileting	86
Intensive toileting	88
Reacting to urgency	89
Diet	89
Reward training	90
Accepting the toilet	90
Glossary	92
Further reading	96

List of Illustrations

Figure 1	The urinary system	5
Figure 2	The bladder outlet, closed and open	6
Figure 3	The lower bowel	8
Figure 4	The frequency of bedwetting	23
Figure 5	Times for a 'staggered waking' schedule	27
Figure 6	Star chart	29
Figure 7	Typical bedwetting alarm	34
Figure 8	'Classical' learning in bedwetting alarm treatment	36
Figure 9	Different types of urine detector mat	45
Figure 10	Simple wet/dry chart	47
Figure 11	Detailed treatment record chart	49
Figure 12	Detector mats across the bed	53
Figure 13	Section of twin mat arrangement in the bed	54
Figure 14	...using pillowcase	54
Figure 15	Typical treatment record graph (actual patient)	58
Figure 16	'Buzzer' box behind furniture (requiring child to rise in order to switch off)	66
Figure 17	'Holding' record chart	71
Figure 18	Record chart for use when 'counting' to reduce approach urgency	73
Figure 19	The daytime 'buzzer'	77
Figure 20	The rectum loaded with a faecal mass	84
Figure 21	Record chart for soiling problems	87

PREFACE

I first became involved in the study and treatment of children's incontinence problems as a newly fledged research worker in 1970, and have been held in my involvement ever since by three factors. Firstly, the extreme personal importance of any incontinence problem to the child and his family. Secondly, the knowledge that something *can* be done, successfully, about the vast majority of children's incontinence problems – despite assurances that it is 'nothing to worry about' and that 'he (or she) will probably grow out of it eventually'. Thirdly – and perhaps most importantly – the fact that many, many children have various routines and treatments used with disappointing results, because knowledge of the techniques and details of their practical use is nowhere near available enough to either parents or professionals. It is also sad (and all too common at the special clinics in which I have worked) to meet a boy or girl who has used the 'buzzer' – a quite effective but difficult treatment described in this book – with disappointing failure because its use was allowed to fall into some of the basic pitfalls of the technique, and the initial explanation and subsequent supervision failed to avoid this.

It is for these same reasons that this book has been written. I hope that it will help to explain what is behind continence and incontinence to both parents and children, assist in deciding whether to seek professional advice, give some ideas for 'self-help' at home, and be a source of useful information when using complex treatment procedures.

Throughout the book, I have tried to stress two main themes. Firstly, the way bladder or bowel control problems can be countered by nothing more mysterious than carefully planned *learning*. Secondly, the importance that, whatever helping technique is tried, its effects should be *recorded* by a simple but consistent chart. Too many treatment efforts are carried out without progress records – yet only by constant recording can treatment techniques be 'fine tuned' while under way, to maximum effectiveness.

ROGER MORGAN
Cambridge, October 1980

ACKNOWLEDGEMENTS

The opinions in this book are my own, but I wish to express my gratitude to those researchers and therapists on whose research I have drawn, from whose experience I have learned, and with whom I have worked. In particular, I am indebted to my colleagues at special incontinence clinics: Dr Gordon Young at Barnet; Dr Keith Turner, Professor Derek Jehu and Professor Martin Herbert when we were together at Leicester and Birmingham; Dr Don Brooksbank and Dr Joan Hay at Chatham, and my current colleagues in Cambridge.

I am also indebted to the many parents and children who have worked so hard on so many courses of treatment, and who have always been so willing to take part in the evaluation of their treatment at research clinics.

Finally, I am indebted especially to my colleagues at the Disabled Living Foundation for their support and sponsorship in the writing of this book.

FOREWORDS

The Trustees of the Disabled Living Foundation gratefully acknowledge grants from the Trustees of the Peter Nathan Charitable Trust, and of a Trust which wishes to remain anonymous, which enabled the manuscript for this book to be prepared. They feel fortunate to have secured the interest of Dr Roger Morgan as author in this relatively undocumented subject, and thank him warmly. They also thank Mr Bill Brennan, the illustrator, for his clear line drawings.

We hope that this book will be useful to both parents and professionals. It is intended to fill a gap, and in view of this both we and the author would be grateful for feedback and comment which would be helpful in improving its usefulness, and which can be incorporated into later editions.

W. M. H. HAMILTON
Chairman of the Trustees
Disabled Living Foundation

While running an Advisory Service on the problems of incontinence I have become aware of the need for some information on the subject of incontinence in children.

This handbook gives an account of the normal working of bladder and bowel, and a detailed analysis of training for continence. It provides a step by step practical guide not only for parents but also for the professionals assisting them.

Dr Roger Morgan has worked for many years with incontinent children and their parents, and he writes with clarity and understanding from a standpoint of great knowledge and experience.

DOROTHY A. MANDELSTAM, MCSP, DipSocSc.
Incontinence Adviser
Disabled Living Foundation

1

INTRODUCTION

There can be few social and physical problems more devastating to one's sense of personal dignity than the inability to exercise full control over bladder or bowel. Few who have not experienced such problems for themselves can fully imagine the feelings of a child who cannot go to sleep at night without the fear that his body will let him down while he is asleep and out of control, so that he awakens in a urine-soaked bed; or of the child who despite desperate efforts at its prevention soils his underclothes with faeces and has to suffer not only personal disgrace and failure, but also the taunts of other children. In the face of such problems, some children not surprisingly react with signs of stress and disturbance as well, while others can only survive by adopting a blasé and devil-may-care attitude. Even in the latter case, it is worth bearing in mind that few children indeed are likely to have become bedwetters, pants-wetters or soilers if they could have avoided it.

The consequences of wetting or soiling for a child are severe. The typical bedwetter tries to keep his problem a secret from all but his closest relatives and friends, and realizes the limitations imposed by his handicap when he does not dare to go to stay with friends, go on school holidays or to Scout or Guide camps. The older child often realizes very acutely the restriction bedwetting places upon jobs which require residential training or residential work – such as nursing, study away from home, or joining the forces. For the day-time wetter or soiler, the problem is there for all to see. Few other children wish to sit next to or make friends with a child who smells of urine or faeces. The parents of an incontinent child owe it to their son or daughter to do their best to understand the problem and to help to overcome it by the best means available.

For a parent, also, the fact that their child wets his bed or soils himself can prove a severely testing problem. Quite apart from a heavy and unpleasant washing load, often day in, day out (an extreme problem in overcrowded living conditions or where washing facilities or buying enough clothing and bedclothing is difficult), other parents and relatives are often critical. Having a child who wets or soils can very easily be taken as some sort of failure as a parent. It is widely recognized that, after excessive crying, wetting and soiling are the most difficult problems that parents may face with young children. Added to this, most parents are unsure whether a wet or soiled older child can, or cannot, 'help it', whether they should sympathize, punish or ignore the problem, and why their particular child or children should seem to be so behind in this respect. It is extremely difficult to deal consistently and rationally with a problem that can be so persistent, off-putting, and frustrating.

Probably because of its fundamental nature, incontinence in children has become the focus of a wealth of folk-lore, and most parents and children involved are likely to come across a wide variety of advice, much of it conflicting and confusing. Opinions differ widely amongst doctors, child psychologists, health visitors and other professionals involved. It is, however, vital to the effectiveness of many forms of management and treatment of incontinence problems in children that parents should have information available on the principles and procedures involved. Without such information, it can become difficult, if not sometimes impossible, to apply and adapt procedures to one's own child and household, and to cope with unexpected setbacks and difficulties. Also, without such information it is difficult to know exactly what to expect, and how soon, when starting to use a particular management or treatment technique. Quite apart from his or her parents, the child who actually has a wetting or soiling problem feels far happier if both the problem and its treatment are explained to him in terms that he can understand – and parents need adequate information before they can pass it on to their child.

The purpose of this book is to provide a source of basic information about the nature and development of bladder and bowel control, and the problems of bedwetting, daytime soiling and daytime wetting in children, describing some of the most common management procedures that may be used by parents as well as the treatments most likely to be advised by doctors, health visitors, or others who may be consulted professionally. Major alternative approaches to the problems are outlined, and one or two common misconceptions discussed. There has been a considerable amount of research into incontinence problems, and the book has been written with this research firmly in mind.

It is intended that the information given should help parents and children to consider and discuss their particular incontinence problem, and to decide whether to seek professional advice. It is also intended to provide background information to help parents to discuss problems and alternative courses of action with the doctor or other person consulted, and to increase the limited amount of information which such a person can give during a brief professional consultation. The information given here may sometimes itself suggest a solution to less severe incontinence problems, but even where professional help is nevertheless needed, it is likely to be more effectively used and will be less frightening to the child if the parents and child are reasonably well-informed about the basic facts. For most people discussing something as personal and distressing as incontinence can be painfully embarrassing, and it is hoped that this book will answer some questions so that they do not have to be asked of anyone else. While aimed primarily at parents, it is hoped that the older boy or girl with a wetting or soiling problem will benefit from reading it, and that those professionally involved with incontinence in children may nevertheless find the book of some use in their work.

One warning must be given; no book can provide a parent with the whole picture and while this book contains some basic information it is not a substitute for the specialized knowledge and practical skills of the doctor. While parents may find the information given useful where giving help to an incontinent child, a doctor should always be consulted where there is a definite incontinence problem. There *may* be a specific issue (perhaps an infection or a particular physical problem) that needs looking into, and most forms of treatment need experienced professional guidance as well as the kind of basic explanation that can be given in a book such as this.

2

Bladder and bowel control—what do they mean?

The structure and working of the bladder

The bladder is the reservoir that holds the urine made by the kidneys until it is emptied out of the body into the toilet or elsewhere. It is an expandable bag with walls of thin muscle (the 'detrusor') which can relax to allow it to grow larger and fill, or contract to squeeze its contents — urine — out on visiting the toilet. It is the muscular wall of the bladder first beginning to contract that gives a person the feeling that he wants to empty his bladder.

The bladder is not like a tank which just fills up until it overflows to result in a wet bed or wet pants, nor is it like a balloon which just stretches as it fills until it can stretch no more and so must empty. It works much harder than that — and can be controlled more easily. Being a bag constructed of muscle, it can make itself larger or smaller by relaxing or contracting, in much the same way as the muscles in one's arm perform their task by relaxing or contracting. While it is filling with urine from the kidneys, the bladder wall relaxes gradually to allow itself to become steadily larger and so contain more urine, without the pressure inside rising very much at all. When it reaches its usual maximum level of filling, it stops relaxing and begins the waves of contractions which normally give rise to the feeling that it must be emptied immediately. When the toilet is reached, or wetting occurs, these contractions become strong enough to empty the bladder.

Each person's bladder has its own usual maximum level of filling (known as the 'functional bladder capacity'), some being very full at this point, but others containing very little indeed. This level is not the point at which the bladder is literally full to bursting, but rather the level at which a particular individual's bladder is used to starting its contractions and so needs to be emptied. Most important is that the usual maximum

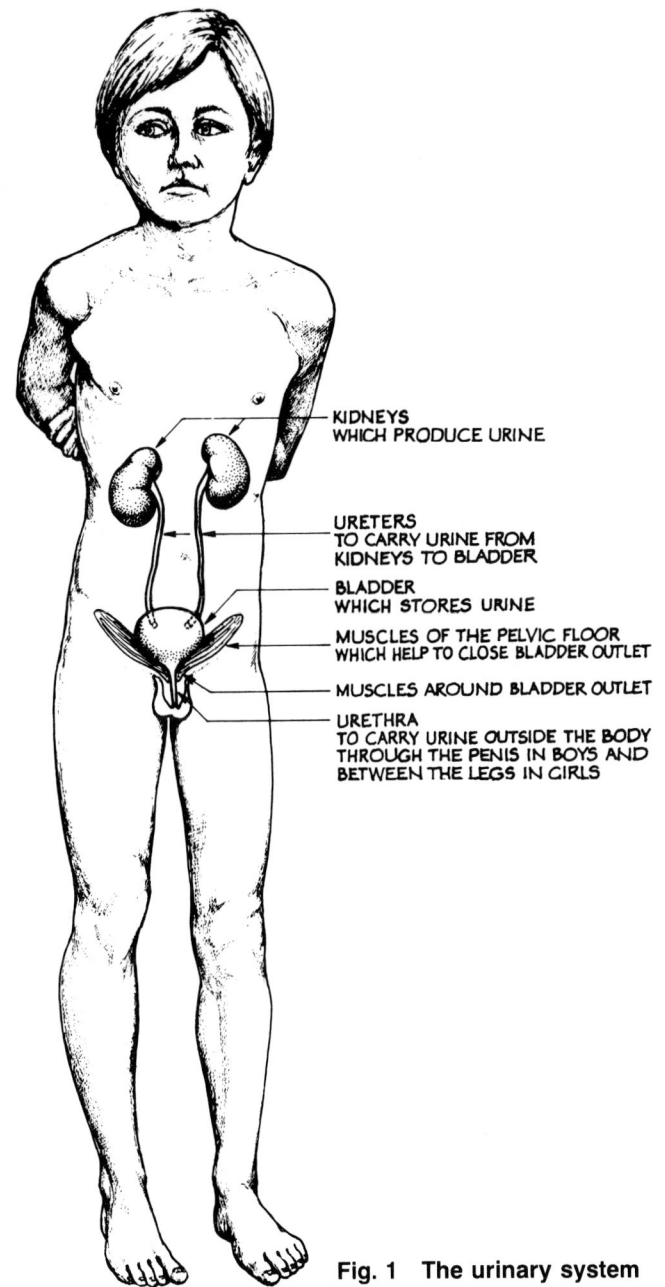

Fig. 1 The urinary system

level of most children's bladders can be changed by changes in habits, as will be described in Chapter 6. Simply drinking less, however, does not often help a child with a wetting problem, since it is one of the ways of encouraging the bladder to adjust itself to a lower maximum level of filling than before.

Figure 1 illustrates the basic structure of the bladder and its inlets and outlet. The urine is carried from the kidneys to the bladder by the two tubes known as ureters, which join the bladder itself at an angle so that when the bladder is very full or is contracting, the ends of the ureters are squeezed shut like valves to prevent urine from being pushed back to the kidneys. The urine leaves the bladder when it is emptied through the tube known as the urethra, which opens on the outside of the body as the front passage between the legs in girls and at the end of the penis in boys. Between emptyings, the bladder outlet is kept closed by a number of factors (closure mechanisms) one of which consists of the muscles of the pelvic floor. These are below the bladder, and the urethra passes through them on its route to the outside (Fig. 2a).

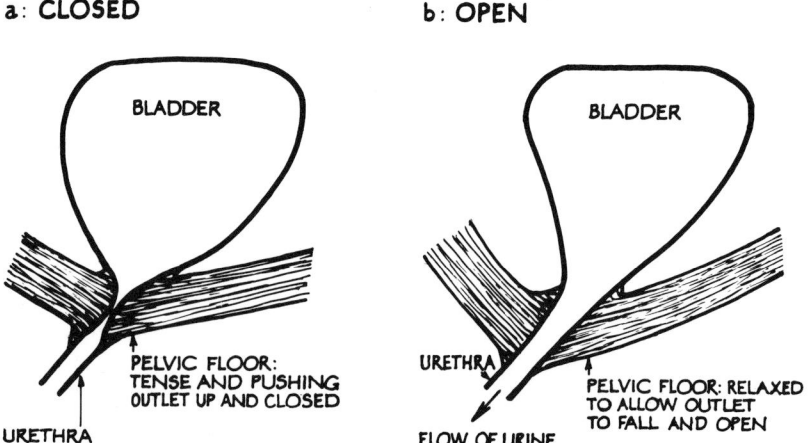

Fig. 2 The bladder outlet, closed and open

When urination begins, the bladder begins to empty, and the pelvic floor muscles relax, which takes the pressure off the urethra and pulls the bladder outlet down and open (see Fig. 2b); at the same time the bladder's contractions push urine through the urethra to emerge outside as the familiar stream or jet of urine. Bladder contractions are encouraged by the downward pull on the bladder wall as the pelvic floor falls downwards, and usually by a general 'push' down onto the bladder by the muscles of the abdomen and diaphragm to trigger the stream. The sensation of urine entering the urethra encourages the stream to continue. We cannot directly control the relaxation or contractions of the bladder wall itself by conscious effort. Like the muscles of the heart or stomach, it is one of the 'automatic' muscles of the body. The muscles we use to control urination are the 'voluntary' muscles of the pelvic floor, abdomen and diaphragm – these muscles being used to 'persuade' the bladder to do what is wanted by pulling and pushing upon it. As we also use these muscles in different ways for many other things, like coughing, sneezing, or laughing, their use in bladder control is complex. It is perhaps more remarkable that so many children achieve bladder control, than that some do not.

On those occasions when the urination is stopped in mid-stream, this is achieved by raising and tightening the pelvic floor to close off the bladder outlet and upper section of urethra, while bladder contractions die down. Leakage of urine from the bladder during coughing, sneezing or laughing can happen if the closure mechanism does not keep the bladder outlet fully 'watertight' despite the extra pressure on the bladder at these times; the structures are so arranged, however, that increased pressure on the bladder at times other than urination (such as during a cough) will usually also put enough pressure on the upper urethra to close it tighter for security whenever the bladder is under extra pressure.

The structure and working of the bowel

The structure of the lower bowel is illustrated in Fig. 3. After passing through the stomach, the food being digested is pushed through the tubes of the small intestine and then the large intestine by the ripple-like waves of contractions in the muscular intestinal wall; the process is known as peristalsis. In its final sections, the large intestine (or colon) runs across the upper front part of the abdomen and then down the left hand front side of the abdomen towards the rectum.

Unlike the colon, with its waves of peristalsis propelling its contents along, the rectum is usually empty, with its walls closed together – it is often described as a 'potential' rather than an 'actual' tube. It is filled at intervals, rather than continuously, with the waste material (faeces) from the digestive process. When a quantity of faeces passes into the rectum, it

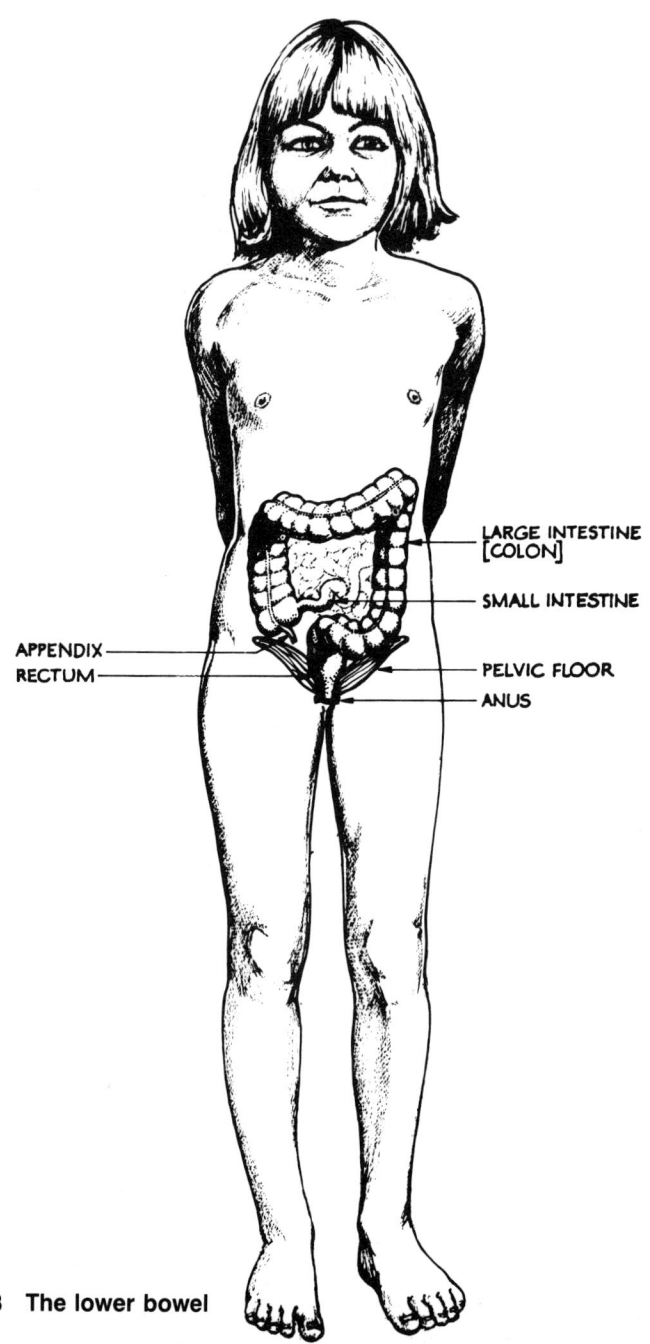

Fig. 3 The lower bowel

stretches to store the material until the toilet is visited and the faeces emptied.

Normally, the filling and emptying into the toilet of the rectum takes place according to a more or less regular routine; this routine can be helped or changed quite markedly by the habits formed in visiting the toilet. The ability of the walls of the rectum to stretch is important to bowel control – by stretching from an empty state, quite large quantities of faeces can be stored in the rectum for short periods until it is convenient to visit the toilet, and it is this stretching of the walls of the rectum that produces the sensation of fullness and the urge to visit the toilet to empty the bowel.

In defaecation, the rectum is emptied through the ring of muscle of the anus. The anus is under voluntary control, and is opened at the start of defaecation, together with a more general relaxation downwards of the pelvic floor muscles. The stretched rectum tends to contract to expel faeces and so collapse to its normally closed-up 'potential tube' state. At the same time, the abdominal and diaphragm muscles are used to place pressure onto the rectum to aid the expulsion of its contents. After defaecation, the anus is closed and the rectum closes in once more.

The basic skills

Many people talk of 'bladder control' or 'bowel control' as if they were single, simple skills. Staying clean and dry however depends as much upon social skills, knowing how to cope under different circumstances (for example, while at school, on a journey, or in a strange place), and the ability to cope with clothing and with different types of toilet, as it does upon bodily 'bladder and bowel' skills. To a very young child, the range of skills needed represents a major field of learning. Even the physical skills concerned with the working of the bladder and bowel themselves are quite numerous. At least eight separate types of skill are needed in order to stay reliably continent – problems in any one can produce difficulties. The eight types of skill are described below:

1 Postponing urination

The ability to 'hold on' to urine, and thus postpone urination, for a reasonable period is essential to staying dry – to avoid urgency or wetting when the toilet or other suitable place is not available, and to allow time to find somewhere to empty the bladder, without rushing or discomfort, once the urge to urinate has been felt. Normal holding ability is sufficient to allow the child to 'last out', without effort or discomfort, between easily convenient and reasonably spaced visits to the toilet, with a sufficient safety margin built in to avoid trouble when under stress or faced with an unusually long wait before the opportunity to urinate.

Postponing urination requires the suppression of overactive contractions of the bladder when relatively empty, and efficiency of the closure mechanism in keeping the bladder outlet closed. The pelvic floor being part of this mechanism, the effectiveness of these muscles is important. Their action is automatic in helping to prevent leakage when coughing, laughing or sneezing, but if inefficient they can be improved by procedures such as those described in Chapter 6. It is remarkable how sensitive these largely automatic functions are to outside influences – it is for instance common for holding ability to be reduced considerably at times of anxiety (such as examinations), when the need to visit the toilet becomes more frequent. At times of extreme fear, holding ability often disappears altogether and wetting occurs – thus the driver or pilot about to crash may wet himself.

Holding ability depends upon the amount of urine which the bladder can hold before it begins to contract, no longer adjusting its own size to accommodate more urine; the 'functional bladder capacity'. It is known that in many who wet the bed, bladder contractions are stronger and more frequent than in other people, and thus this point is reached with relatively little urine in the bladder. In many children with a daytime problem, the pelvic floor muscles too easily allow the bladder outlet to open slightly – particularly when under the physical stress of actions such as coughing. This reduces holding ability, partly by allowing urine to leak out and thus wetting to occur, and partly because once urine enters the urethra (see Fig. 1) a sensation of urgency is felt and urination will tend to continue.

2 Keeping the rectum empty

Whereas holding urine, within reasonable limits, is important to bladder control, bowel control requires that the rectum (see Fig. 3) is normally kept empty, and is emptied by defaecation shortly after the urge to defaecate is felt. This requires firstly the habit of *not* holding on to faeces for long periods after the urge to defaecate, and secondly the establishment of regular bowel function (in which the rectum fills at generally

BLADDER AND BOWEL CONTROL

predictable intervals, convenient for subsequent defaecation) through regularity of toilet visits.

3 Perceiving the need to empty

Both bladder and bowel control require that the individual receives and responds to the urge to empty — the urge to urinate arising from bladder contractions and to defaecate from the filling and stretching of the rectum. Different individuals actually feel quite different sensations of urgency to urinate, in different parts of the body. Under normal circumstances the body learns to perceive urgency early enough for holding ability to last until a toilet is reached, but when a toilet or other suitable place cannot be reached within the normal 'holding time' (as perhaps on a journey or during certain school activities), holding ability can run out and wetting occurs.

Our perception of urgency, like many other continence skills, is remarkably sensitive to outside influences. Urgency is often suppressed when other people are present while urination is attempted (such as in hospital wards), it can be reduced or not felt when a child is engrossed in some distracting activity, and it can be triggered or intensified by thinking about visiting the toilet. The approach to and sight of a toilet have the capacity in most of us to trigger or increase urgency. It is a common experience for urgency to increase dramatically as the toilet is approached, particularly if one is near the limits of one's holding ability, so that sometimes one 'only just makes it'. This urgency-response of the bladder's control mechanisms when near a toilet serves the purpose of a reminder to urinate if necessary when the opportunity is there.

4 Starting the urine stream

Humans are almost the only animal species capable of voluntarily starting the process of emptying the bladder when it is less than full. The skill is complex, involving as already described the co-ordinated use of the pelvic floor, abdominal and diaphragm muscles. The factors that affect urgency will also affect ability to start the urine stream. In addition, the skill is affected by anything that affects the main muscle groups involved. Thus it is often found that passing urine is difficult, and sometimes not possible without medical help, shortly after an abdominal operation has temporarily impaired the ability to place pressure on the bladder by contracting abdominal and diaphragm muscles.

The very young child empties his bladder when it is full (ie at its functional capacity), but as he grows older the practice of normal bladder control requires that he develop increased sophistication in the initiation of the urine stream at lower levels than this, so that he can make use of toilets when available. Fortunately, it is rare for a child to experience difficulty in initiating the stream of urine voluntarily.

5 Starting defaecation

Bowel control relies heavily upon the regular working of the lower bowel. A key to the establishment of regular and controllable bowel function is the establishment of regular defaecation, encouraging a comparable regularity in the periodic filling of the rectum.

Initiating defaecation, just as initiating urination, requires the effective co-ordinated use of pelvic floor, abdominal and diaphragm muscles to put pressure where it is needed and to allow free passage for the faeces to be ejected. In addition the anus must be relaxed to open the outlet of the rectum, the anus being an integral part of the larger pelvic floor.

Defaecation, as with the skills of bladder control, can be affected by a person's surroundings, and is for instance easily inhibited by the presence of other people. It can also be disrupted by physical factors. Constipation can render expulsion of the large and hard mass of faeces difficult, requiring high pressures on the rectum and a widely stretched anus. Any small split in the anus, or piles, can hinder defaecation by making it painful.

6 Monitoring and responding while asleep

Problems of bowel control at night are very rare, the rectum's filling and need to empty occurring usually during the daytime. Problems of bladder control, and thus bedwetting are however, very common. The effectiveness of the body's monitoring of the state of the bladder during sleep is central to a child's remaining dry at night. Where holding ability is low, so that the bladder requires emptying during the night, it is particularly important that the monitoring system should arouse the child early enough and completely enough for the toilet to be visited. As the bladders of bedwetting children are liable to frequent contractions throughout the night, it is all the more important that awaking from sleep should occur when these contractions begin to build up to a peak that is likely to result in wetting.

Most people assume that deep sleep is a cause of bedwetting, because it might bring poor bladder monitoring at night. This is not the case, however, as research studies have shown that bedwetting occurs at various stages and levels of sleep, and not solely at the deepest. At the time of wetting, the problem is that the body is not handling its bladder signals correctly, not that it is too deeply asleep. Indeed, it is often only just below the level of wakefulness that wetting happens, regardless of whether the child is a 'deep sleeper' or not.

Most children's bodies do automatically monitor and respond to bladder contractions, but in those who wet the bed, the monitoring, or the body's response to it, is not strong enough. Most children will move about in bed just before they wet, and their brain becomes more active than during normal sleep, this activity becoming greater as the child grows older. It may become strong enough to avoid bedwetting with increasing age alone in some children, who thus grow out of the problem. In some children the monitoring and response is stronger than that producing simply restlessness and possibly a toilet dream, but still not strong enough to wake the child up completely. Such children may partially awake, and without being conscious enough to visit the toilet properly, automatically perform only part of the procedure – urinating on the carpet or in some odd corner, or even preparing to go to school. These odd actions are not usually deliberate, but the result of incomplete waking. The process of holding on and waking to find the toilet is a complex chain of events that needs plenty of notice from the monitoring system.

A child cannot improve the sleep-monitoring of his (probably particularly active) bladder simply by trying or being told to do so. Nevertheless, the monitoring process does change in different circumstances. Monitoring of the bladder when sleeping in unfamiliar circumstances away from home tends to be more efficient, just as the sounds in and outside an unfamiliar bedroom are noticed more. Thus the majority of bedwetting children wet less when staying with relatives, on holiday, or even in hospital. A child's body can be trained by the enuresis alarm (described in Chapters 4 and 5) to monitor the bladder more efficiently, selecting signals concerning contractions from the bladder for special attention. Signals which the brain has learned are important can produce a response even during the unconsciousness of sleep; the brain will for instance react during sleep to a tape recording of one's name, but not to the equally loud but meaningless sound of the same tape recording played backwards.

7 Knowing when and where to 'go'

Parents who have ever wondered for a moment what to do with a bidet will appreciate how a very young child feels when faced with different kinds of toilet. He must learn first that it is his pot, and not the room it is in or anything else, that is his 'go-ahead' for urination or defaecation. Then he must learn that various toilets and other places can be used. There are however many confusions – some toilets are reserved for 'staff' or one sex only; chemical closets, campsite toilets in the ground, and some foreign toilets are very different from the pot or toilet at home. There are some places that can be used sometimes but not at others – thus one can go behind a tree when away from a toilet, but not when it is just outside a house or near a toilet; boys must learn that one does not urinate in public – except in a gentlemen's public lavatory. Knowing when and where one may go is not inborn, but a skill that has to be acquired when very young.

8 Coping with clothing, cleaning and toilet equipment

Going to the toilet without help demands a range of supplementary 'coping' skills in addition to bladder and bowel control.

With any complicated skill, those who can do it will tend to forget how many separate elements it has. The adult can easily think of 'going to the toilet' as if it were a single act, just as the experienced car driver can think of driving off in the car as a single act, forgetting the separate elements of using the ignition, throttle, clutch, gear, steering, brake and signalling controls. The child does not just 'visit the toilet' – after feeling the urge to go, he must hold on while he finds the right time to go and reaches the toilet, he must open and close doors as necessary, raise or lower a lavatory seat, adjust his clothing as needed, stand or sit in the right position (depending on sex) to avoid making a mess (boys needing to decide whether to stand or sit, and to 'aim' straight when urinating), cleanse as necessary, readjust clothing, flush the toilet (flushing systems varying enormously, often being difficult to use and requiring considerable strength), wash hands, and return without being accidentally wet, soiled, or improperly dressed.

Learning the skills – taught or just acquired?

Before each of the skills described can be used to help the child to remain clean and dry two conditions must be met. Firstly, the body must have developed sufficiently for it to be possible for the muscles and nervous system to perform the necessary actions. Secondly, the physical skills must be developed and moulded through a process of learning, involving the association of one thing with another, the shaping of actions and reactions according to their pleasant or unpleasant consequences, and the imitation of examples set by others.

Clearly, most of the skills of continence involve learning by the child. 'Holding' actions must become associated with first signals of urgency from bladder or bowel, encouraged by the avoidance of unpleasant consequences such as becoming dirty or wet and cold, and by giving pleasant consequences such as praise for toileting rather than having an 'accident'. One reason for boys having more incontinence problems than girls is probably that boys' skins are less sensitive to the unpleasantness of being wet and cold, one factor in this learning. The efficient use of the pelvic floor in holding on and in starting urination and defaecation must be learned, as must the use of the pelvic floor, abdominal and diaphragm muscles in different ways to achieve different results. The link between strong bladder contractions while asleep and the twin reactions of holding on and waking up must also be learned.

The question arises as to whether this learning needs to be *taught* to the child, or whether it will happen quite naturally. A number of points may be made in answer. Firstly, some of the learning – such as the co-ordination of various internal muscles – is so complex that no parent could possibly teach it to a child, any more than one could teach a child what he must do to raise his arm. These bodily skills are learned without help; it is interesting to note that many children show that they have learned, without being taught, that lifting the pelvic floor reduces urgency, when they press it upwards by sitting on a heel or a hard edge. Secondly, a large proportion of the necessary learning is known to occur quite naturally, without teaching, provided that all normal opportunities for learning and practice are available. Thirdly, some of the learning does require a helping hand and encouragement, although formal teaching or training would be more than is needed for most children. Thus parents need to help introduce a child to the idea of a pot or toilet, and to praise success at toileting and at holding urine.

The learning of continence is very similar to learning to speak. In learning speech, the complex bodily movements to produce the sounds are learned but cannot be taught by the average parent; opportunity to hear and practise speech is needed, praise for success is given, and some help is needed with the unfamiliar.

All learning can be held back or broken up, even when complete, by serious stress, and learning of bladder and bowel control is no exception. Children who suffer serious stress when aged 2 to 3 years, while they are acquiring continence, are often likely to have difficulties with bladder or bowel control. In addition, it should be noted that the skills of continence are not equally easy for all children, any more than the skills of playing the piano are equally easy for all, and they are sufficiently difficult for some children to prevent their normal development. Some children are also more sensitive to the disrupting effects of stress than are others.

Most readers of this book will have come across either the failure or breakdown of bladder or bowel control. Stress or difficulty, which can be inherited, in the particular skills concerned in continence may well be involved, and intensive training in the problematic skills as described in later chapters is required to remedy the situation. However, failure or breakdown of continence is not likely to result from any lack of formal toilet training in early childhood.

Toilet training and its effects

Having noted that the most useful form of toilet training is likely to consist of a 'helping hand' with opportunities, guidance and praise, rather than any kind of formal training course, it is also worth noting that most parents start too early and are probably too formal over toilet training. A major British research study of child upbringing reported that one in five mothers had started 'training' before their children were two months old, two thirds by eight months, and over eight out of ten by the first birthday. For most children, training at any time in the first year is asking too much of the child's physical maturity.

The more common training techniques are outlined below:

1 Daytime 'potting'

Potting the child during the day is the most common form of toilet training. However, its effect is overrated; research studies have found it to have little beneficial effect upon either daytime or night-time wetting, and if it becomes a source of stress and conflict between parents and child (as it can easily do) it can even slow down the learning of continence. Potting does however help with bowel control to some extent, although children who are not 'potted' soon catch up with those who are.

BLADDER AND BOWEL CONTROL

From our earlier analysis of the various elements of continence it is clear that learning to produce urine or faeces in the pot is a relatively small part of the overall skill of continence. Potting gives a temporary lead in bowel control because it helps to keep the rectum in its normal empty state, in which it is most sensitive to the stretch-effect of faeces entering. Because the bladder, however, being quite a different structure, needs to become adjusted to holding urine rather than frequently emptying, emptying it into a pot has little effect on holding ability. It does probably help however in learning to start urinating at will, and in learning one acceptable place in which to urinate.

Potting is likely to be helpful to some extent, but is a great deal of effort for relatively little gain, and children not 'potted' will usually do just as well in the long run.

2 Night-time 'potting'

Many parents 'lift' or wake their children, often when they come to bed themselves, to urinate in the toilet. Again, such a potting procedure can help, but it is much effort for little benefit in many cases. It is a procedure many parents seen with their children at incontinence clinics have been following without results for years. If night potting has been tried for six months without results, it is unlikely to be worth continuing. The child is probably either not yet sufficiently mature physically for night-time control, or the technique is not an effective one for him. It may be tried again, for a similar period, a year or so later.

The problem with night potting is that while it does at least mean some urine in the toilet rather than the bed, it does not teach or train the child to develop his or her own bodily control. He does not learn to associate waking up with the feeling of a full bladder, because his bladder is unlikely to be full just at the point his parents lift or wake him. Night potting can produce odd effects on rare occasions; I have come across children at clinics who have learned to empty their bladders when they hear someone approaching at night, because they have learned to associate these events. Others, if not potted, will wet at what has become the usual time, thus relying on parental help rather than body control to stay dry. These odd effects can be reduced by night potting at irregular times and avoiding a similar routine each night — so that it does not encourage regular habits of reliance and wetting.

3 Encouragement and praise

Praising a child for success, immediately and for even small steps of progress, is one of the best forms of help a parent can give. It is not a training 'routine' but a matter of looking out for each small step and praising for it. It encourages toilet control in exactly the same way as it assists walking when first steps are noticed and praised, or talking when first words are picked out and responded to. Much research into toilet training and the learning of other skills has demonstrated how powerful immediate praise for small steps of progress can be, and it is important to note that all learning is more efficient when it is encouraged and reinforced by praise. Progress should be looked for in each of the basic skills already described, not just in 'producing' in the pot. To praise a child for holding urine and staying dry, even for short periods at first, is equally important.

4 Punishment

Many parents punish children for 'accidents', at the same time as they are following a potting routine. Accidents must be expected, however, and while praise for success effectively 'seals' the learning in a little more firmly each time, punishment of failures does less to encourage continence. Where an 'accident' is simply a matter of not enough skill, punishment is probably useless; and it is worth remembering, when a child soils or wets just after refusing an opportunity to 'go', that knowing when you need to go is a skill to be learned like the others.

5 Changes in circumstances

Where a child has almost achieved control, a major change like coming out of nappies, having 'grown-up' clothes or pyjamas, or changing beds, will often be enough to tip the balance into full control. The danger of course is in making such a change when the child is not ready, and then being disappointed when he fails to achieve success.

6 Restricting fluids

Fluids should not be restricted as a toilet training technique. The less-full bladder is not likely to empty less, other than immediately after the start of fluid restrictions. All that happens is that the functional capacity of the bladder (as already described) reduces, so that the bladder performs all its usual urgency and emptying, but at a lower level of filling than before. Holding ability, which is central to bladder control, is thus impaired and bladder control actually reduced by fluid restriction.

7 Demonstration

Children need to learn how to cope with toilets and clothing, and much of this is learned by watching others and simply by being shown what to do. Being shown each stage of what to do, with less help as the child begins to pick up the skill for himself, and with praise to seal in any progress made, is as powerful a form of toilet training as most children need or can benefit from.

Some special intensive 'programmes' of toilet training are now available in published form. These are highly formal procedures, usually based on the idea of immediate and intensive praise for success and perhaps remedial training for failures. They are perhaps reasonably seen as a concentrated focusing of commonsense and effective techniques to accelerate the natural learning of continence. Some use devices worn in the underclothes to signal wetting — simply to aid parents in praising holding and in effect to stop wetting in its tracks while the child is taken to the toilet. Another, designed by Dr Azrin and his colleagues in America (see Further Reading p.96) involves increased drinking, very frequent toileting, extensive praise for both production in the toilet and for remaining clean and dry, and prolonged practice of toileting, with reprimands for accidents. Guidance in dressing and adjusting clothing is included.

Such intensive training certainly has a place (where for instance only intensive training can help a handicapped child, or where for some reason it is more than usually important for a child to become continent quickly), but it demands very great effort and determination on the part of all concerned, and has to be applied strictly as designed — which not all parents find easy or pleasant. If one wishes to use such a programme, it is easier, and likely to be more effective, if it is professionally supervised.

Other aids are also on the market, including a pot which plays a tune when filled. This is another variation on the theme of praise for success — although again it must be said that continence involves learning far more than production in the pot. It is also an expensive way of giving a praising reaction — parents can praise or reward equally effectively themselves.

Conclusion — encouraging continence

The key words in toilet training are opportunity, encouragement and praise. One should not expect anything to happen towards becoming clean and dry until around the middle of the second year of life (much later than most parents start trying to toilet train), when the first signs occur indicating that the child's bodily awareness and control are beginning to develop towards continence. These first signs (which do not need to be taught) are the child showing awareness that urination or defaecation are about to happen, perhaps clutching at himself and holding urine for just a moment, and first showing a dislike of being wet or soiled. At this point, introduction to the idea of a pot (but not necessarily regular potting), and opportunity to use it at the right time, are appropriate. Parents should notice any step, however small, in each of the toileting skills already described, praising and perhaps occasionally rewarding their child for steps of progress, but expecting setbacks. No-one suddenly acquires full competence in any skill. Success at holding and coping with clothing should be noticed and praised, just as much as successful urination or bowel movements in the pot. At an appropriate point, nappies need to be left off for a period — and accidents at this changeover are inevitable. In the case of a mentally handicapped child, a systematic 'programme' of encouragement and praise has been found effective for many, as described in Chapter 6.

Toilet training is taken too seriously by most — the majority of children, with a 'helping hand' as just outlined, will become clean and dry as naturally as they learn to speak, and children not 'trained' become just as continent as those who are. Lack of formal toilet training does not cause wetting or soiling, and the child with a wetting or soiling problem would probably have had the same problem regardless of his parents training or not training him.

3

The problem of bedwetting

Nature and frequency

Whether a bed is wet or not is relatively easy to determine. Whether a particular child should be considered a bedwetter is, however, not so clear. How often wetting happens, how long wetting continues, and the child's age must all be taken into account. Bedwetting (or 'nocturnal enuresis') may be defined as persistent and frequent urination during sleep, at an age at which a greater degree of night-time bladder control is considered to be normal. Many children (and not a few adults) have the occasional wet bed and in most cases this need be of little concern. The 'occasional accident' may be regarded as becoming 'bedwetting' when it is frequent and persistent enough to constitute a problem.

Deliberate wetting

Very many parents wonder whether perhaps the bedwetting child is just basically 'lazy' and could be dry if he wished. This however is extremely unlikely to be the case — the number of children who regularly but deliberately wet the bed when awake is almost negligible.

Many parents will have noticed that their usually bedwetting child tends to wet less, or not at all, when sleeping away from home — on holiday, perhaps, or with relatives. It is all too easy to interpret this as evidence of some element of choice by the child in whether or not to be wet. This is however not the case. Wetting behaviour is in fact very, and quite automatically, sensitive to changes; just as one is more aware and easily awoken by outside sounds when sleeping in unfamiliar surroundings, so one is also most aware of, and easily woken by, the functioning of one's own body. The body's awareness of bladder activity increases when sleeping in unusual circumstances — as if the brain is more actively on 'sentry duty' when asleep away from home. It is surprising, but common, that a bedwetting child may wet less even when under the stress of being in hospital.

How many children wet the bed?

Bedwetting becomes less frequent among older children. The decrease in numbers of bedwetters with increasing age is greatest amongst younger children. There is no sudden tendency to become dry at puberty. If one were to take a hundred bedwetting children aged between 5 and 19, one would expect between 13 and 16 of them to become dry within a year, simply through growing older and without any special treatment.

The number of children one would define as bedwetters depends upon the frequency of wetting one picks as constituting 'bedwetting' rather than 'occasional accidents'. However, when research studies adopting various definitions are put together, the incidence of frequent and persistent bedwetting may be expected to be approximately 11% at the age of five, 7% at the age of seven, 5% at ten, and between 1 and 2% amongst those over fifteen – including adults. These figures are illustrated in Fig. 4. This frequency is higher than most children, and many parents, realize; it is worth saying to a ten year old worried at his bedwetting that even though he may not know about it, he is unlikely to be the only one with the problem even amongst his own classmates at school.

Sex ratio

Approximately twice as many boys as girls have a bedwetting problem. There are many theories as to why this is so; the one already mentioned as probable being that boys' skins are rather less sensitive to the feelings of being wet and cold, which plays a part in the natural learning of bladder control.

Social class

Fewer children of 'professional' families tend to have a bedwetting problem than the children of unskilled parents. This difference is particularly marked amongst older children and amongst bedwetting girls.

The beginning of the problem

Between eight and nine out of ten bedwetting children (and most adult enuretics) are lifelong (or 'primary') bedwetters, never having been dry for a significant period. Those who lose their night-time bladder control

THE PROBLEM OF BEDWETTING

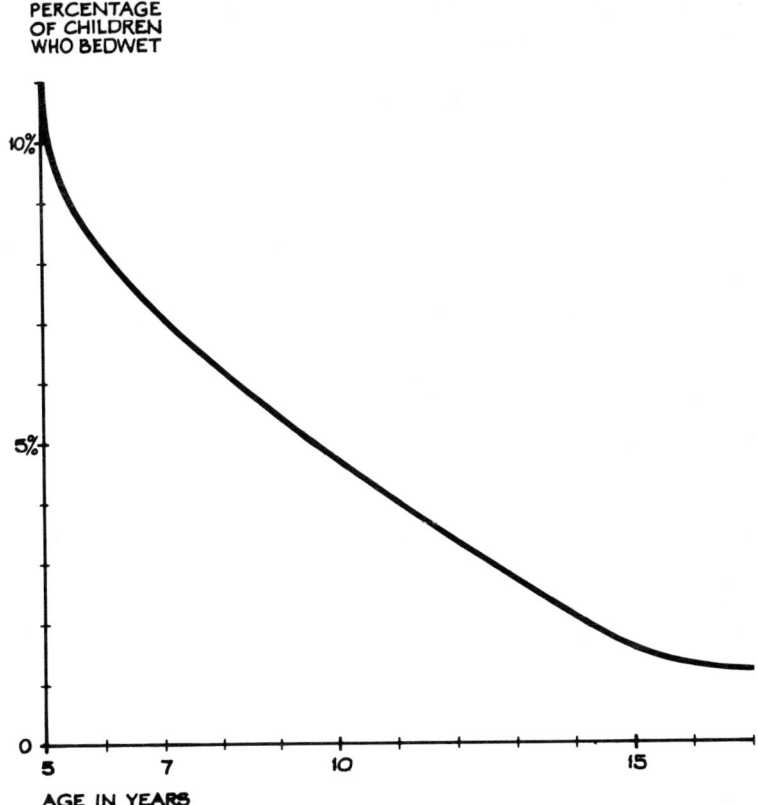

Fig. 4 The frequency of bedwetting

after a reasonable period of control are often termed 'secondary' bedwetters. However, there is little agreement on how long a 'reasonable period' of control is, and the child who has never been consistently dry has basically the same problem as the child who has lost his previous control, even after a number of years. The one has found control hard to achieve, the other has only just managed to achieve it but not hold onto it, perhaps in the face of some change or stress. Both are likely to respond to the same treatments in the same way.

Bedwetting in families

Problems of bladder control tend to run in families, and there is evidence that difficulty in gaining or holding on to bladder control can to some extent be inherited. Some parents of bedwetters will therefore remember having the same problem themselves in their own childhood, or will come across it in other children of the family or among relatives. It seems that bladder control problems must be expected amongst some members, and in each generation, of families where bladder control happens to be a particularly problematic skill.

The origins of bedwetting

It is probable that any one child's bedwetting has a number of causes contributing to it, rather than being produced by any single, easily identifiable cause. The following list gives the more common factors that one may come across:

Emotional stress. Both failure to gain full bladder control in the first place, and its loss once gained, are often linked to some major change or stress in the child's life. There is research evidence that stresses and anxieties in the third or fourth year of life may result in bedwetting, and stresses such as family breakdown, problems at school, moving house, or the birth of a new brother or sister can break up bladder control that has already been gained. The same stresses will not trigger bedwetting in all children, but some children are particularly sensitive to certain forms of stress, and bladder control is a particularly difficult and insecure skill for some children.

Once bladder control has been disrupted, it may return naturally with time – but very often special treatment will be necessary to restore it. Bedwetting is of course in itself a source of anxiety and stress, which can create a vicious circle by hindering the learning necessary to regain the skills of control. The stress that prevented control or triggered bedwetting has very often long passed – even a brief stress at the age of two or three can leave a child wetting perhaps for years, and the 'secondary' bedwetting that starts after a period of dryness can remain long after any triggering stress has passed and been forgotten. Bedwetting tends to be more persistent where there are family difficulties.

Individual differences. There are great differences, partly inherited, between children in the ease with which they acquire and keep bladder control. For some, full and permanent control seems to emerge quickly and effortlessly, whereas others have serious problems. Bedwetting can be due to little more than the fact that a child happens to find the skills of control difficult. Children differ in the ease with which they learn complex physical skills like swimming or riding a bicycle, and they differ just as much with other physical skills like bladder or bowel control.

Infection. Bedwetting can be triggered by an infection in the urinary system (some 16% of children with such infection wet the bed), and wetting in its turn increases the possibility of an infection occurring. This is particularly so in girls, although the majority of bedwetters are nevertheless infection-free. About one in twenty bedwetting girls may be expected to have infection. Because of the infection risk, a doctor should be consulted in all cases of persistent wetting. He is able to check for infection by sending a urine sample to be examined at the laboratory. Any infection found can usually be cured simply through a course of antibiotic tablets. Infections need to be treated as problems in their own right, and removing an infection will help to relieve the wetting. However, specific treatment of the wetting as well is still needed in about 70% of bedwetting children with an infection. Usually the wetting and antibiotic treatments can take place at the same time.

Abnormalities. Very few cases of bedwetting are caused by any physical abnormality – far fewer than most parents and children might fear. A doctor can and should be asked to check a bedwetting child physically, which will in the vast majority of cases result in the reassurance that all is well, but will also pick up the rare case in which there may be something physically wrong which may need further investigation and perhaps a special form of treatment. Where a minor physical abnormality is found, it may nevertheless be that one of the basic treatments for bedwetting will still improve bladder control to some extent. Contrary to popular belief, bedwetting in boys has nothing to do with whether or not the boy has been circumcised, and is not caused by undescended testicles.

Many people regard bedwetting as caused by a 'weak bladder'. This idea does not however explain a great deal, as the crucial factor in the bladder's holding ability is its functional capacity (the level of filling at which contractions and urgency begin), which is capable of quite marked change. This has little to do with 'strength' or 'weakness' of the bladder as an organ. Weakness of the pelvic floor muscles between the legs would however be important, as it may result in failure to keep the bladder outlet raised and closed.

Deep sleep. Contrary to the almost universal belief, bedwetting has virtually nothing to do with deep sleep. Research has established that bedwetting happens at all stages and depths of sleep (except for dreaming sleep), not just the deepest. The 'toilet dreams' experienced by some children, in which they dream they are at the toilet when actually wetting in the bed, are not dreams which lead to urination, but the other way round — the dream is triggered by a wetting which has failed to waken the child, just 'registering' in his consciousness sufficiently to affect his dreaming. Not surprisingly, drugs aimed at nothing more than lightening sleep have not proved effective treatments for bedwetting.

Emotional disturbance. Bedwetting is regarded by some as an expression of some deep emotional disturbance, any treatment therefore being aimed at the disturbance that is assumed to be there, rather than at the bedwetting as such. It is sometimes described as a 'safety valve' for psychological disturbance.

It is certainly true that more bedwetters than dry children have various emotional problems. However, three points are worth making on this issue: firstly, although more bedwetters than others may have emotional problems, most bedwetters are nevertheless psychologically completely normal. Secondly, it is not surprising that bedwetting and emotional problems come together in some children, since both can be caused by the same factors — such as family stresses. Thirdly, bedwetting in itself is a source of stress which can actually cause emotional problems.

It does not therefore seem true to consider a child as 'disturbed' simply because he wets the bed. One should not assume that bedwetting in some way *needs* to be there to serve as a safety valve. Some people worry that if bedwetting itself is cured by a specific form of treatment, something else may go wrong — perhaps another problem would emerge to take the place of the 'safety valve' that has been removed. Careful research into the subject has however clearly shown that no such substitute problem does emerge when bedwetting is treated directly. Bedwetting can be treated directly as a problem no more nor less than poor bladder control, without the fear that it may be an emotional safety valve, or that its removal will affect anything else.

Common ways of helping the bedwetting child

Many parents coping with a bedwetting problem will have come across

THE PROBLEM OF BEDWETTING

one or more of the following approaches, some based on toilet training strategies already described:

Lifting. Waking the child at night to visit the toilet has been noted in Chapter 2 as a common but not highly effective form of toilet training. Parents of older bedwetters have often tried lifting, without results, for a number of years. As we have already seen, lifting rarely improves control, even if it does keep some urine from the bed, and it can teach a child to rely on being woken — and even (although rarely) to wet automatically in response to household sounds. As suggested for toilet training, a staggered timing and non-routine programme of lifting is worth trying, but is not likely to improve bladder control if it has not done so within six months. Possible times of waking for a 'staggered waking' routine are given in Fig. 5.

Day	*Time since bedtime that the child should be woken*
1	1 HOUR
2	3 HOURS
3	1½ HOURS
4	4 HOURS
5	2 HOURS
6	3½ HOURS
7	2½ HOURS
(then repeat)	

Fig. 5   Times for a 'staggered waking' schedule

Punishment. Punishing a child for wetting the bed is not likely to improve matters. It is understandable that parents may lose patience at times — but it does not help. Praising or rewarding successes has more effect in the development of bladder control (or any other skill for that matter) than punishing mistakes or failures.

The different effects of praise and punishment for a child learning bladder control are rather like those that might be experienced by a learner driver learning to change gear. He is more likely to succeed if smooth gear-changes are noticed and praised, while being criticized for jerky or noisy changes is unlikely to help.

Rewards. As we have said, rewarding success will help the development of bladder control both in older children and during the development of control in infancy. By keeping a record of wet and dry nights, any progress can be noticed (gradual progress is often unnoticed without some form of record). Rewarding success is more effective than punishing failures, and is most effective if it is immediate and based on quite small steps forward (thus it is better to reward for each dry night, or each waking to visit the toilet, rather than to arrange something like a bicycle as a reward for a long period dry). Praise is as good a reward as any, but the occasional tangible reward, as a celebration of progress made, is fine.

It is important to stress that the fact that rewards can improve learning does *not* imply that a child could 'do it if he tried'. All learning is more efficient if rewarded for successes, and it is worth remembering that even animals can learn better when praised or rewarded.

In America there has been some promising development of the highly intensive reward and punishment training programme as a treatment for bedwetting similar to the programme already referred to under toilet training. It is however early days for this technique to be fully tested and available in this country.

Star charts. A record of wet and dry nights can be converted into a reward system, especially for the younger child, by using it as a star chart on which he can place stick on stars for dry nights (see Fig. 6). The reward effect of stars can be reinforced with praise and with the occasional 'back-up' tangible reward. Even with the older child, a straightforward wet and dry chart (as illustrated in Fig. 10, p.47) can have a positive effect if used to pinpoint successes.

Restricting fluids. From the previous discussion of the way in which the bladder functions (see p.4), it is clear that fluid restriction as a way of trying to control bedwetting is based on a misconception, and does not help. Cutting down on fluids can, unfortunately, appear to help at first – but only until the bladder begins to adjust to the lower intake, after which restriction can reduce control by reducing holding ability. A bedwetting child should be allowed to drink when thirsty, even if this is

THE PROBLEM OF BEDWETTING

A STAR CHART

Name ....

Starting Date ....

	WEEKS											
	1	2	3	4	5	6	7	8	9	10	11	12
MONDAY												
TUESDAY												
WEDNESDAY												
THURSDAY												
FRIDAY												
SATURDAY												
SUNDAY												

Put a "W" for a Wet night
Draw or stick on a Star for a Dry night

Fig. 6 Star chart

just before bed. As will be seen in Chapters 5 and 6, fluid *increase* rather than fluid *reduction* forms a part of some treatment techniques in order to improve holding capacity.

Common forms of treatment

Once advice has been sought from a doctor or other professional person about bedwetting, one of the following basic courses of action is likely to be advised. Naturally, other ways of coping or helping may be suggested, and different children may need different forms of help, but the approaches outlined below are the most common and the most researched.

Before one's visit to seek professional advice for a wetting or soiling problem, it is helpful to keep a record of wet and dry nights, as, unless wetting is every night without exception, it is very common for one's estimate of wetting frequency to be inaccurate. Also, as stressed throughout this book, a record is indispensable in checking progress, and a record of the position before treatment is a very useful basis for comparison. A chart of the type illustrated in Fig. 10 is simple and helpful.

Reassurance. 'Reassurance' has been included here because it is very often the main help offered by a doctor, particularly for bedwetting in a fairly young child. To know that there is nothing physically wrong, and that there are no signs of infection, are very important and reassuring results of consulting a doctor, and it is true that most bedwetters will 'grow out' of the problem eventually. Between 13 and 16 per cent do in each year. However, some children may take years to do so, and thus it is worth discussing some form of positive treatment where bedwetting is causing distress, particularly in an older child.

Drug treatments. The use of tablets or medicines is the most common form of positive treatment. A number of different types of medication is available, some drugs being available in both tablet and medicine form. Commonly used drugs are Tofranil, Tyrimide, Tryptizol and Cetiprin. Many of the drugs used work on the principle of 'dampening down' the sensitivity and activity of the bladder, reducing its tendency to contract too quickly and actively once it reaches the first stages of urgency, and also increasing its functional capacity — and thus the child's holding ability. A number of these drugs are also used in the treatment of other and often quite different problems — some, for example, are also used for the treatment of depression in adults. Drugs just to lighten sleep are not very often used, as deep sleep is not usually the problem. In all cases, drugs used to treat bedwetting should be used strictly in accordance with the doctor's instructions — like any drugs, a higher dosage than has been prescribed can be dangerous.

Because there is a number of drugs that might be suitable, it is well worth recording progress with any that are prescribed, and visiting the doctor again to ask his advice on a possible change if a particular drug does not appear to be working.

There is one drawback with drug treatments for bedwetting, whichever drug is used. That is the tendency for wetting to start again once the tablets or medicine has been stopped. This is mainly because the drugs do not directly train the body to increase control, nor have a permanent 'dampening down' effect on the bladder after being stopped. They may however in some cases reduce the problem while the body's own control develops enough to take over, and they can reduce the unhelpful stress and anxiety of continued wetting. Drugs may be expected to produce a lasting cure in about one in five cases – and are useful in the short term in suppressing wetting for a period when it matters more than usually (perhaps reducing wet nights on holiday or at times of stress). They are certainly useful, even if they may not effect permanent bladder control, when parents feel they cannot cope with continued wetting without seriously losing their temper and ability to stay sympathetic. Drug treatment also has the distinct advantage that it is easier and not stressful to use compared with the more effective but very demanding 'buzzer' treatment described in later chapters.

Psychotherapy. As has already been discussed, although opinions differ widely on whether bedwetting is linked to emotional disturbance, it seems safe and effective to treat bedwetting as a problem on its own, without fear of causing problems by removing some kind of 'safety valve' from the child.

Psychotherapy treatments, involving play therapy or talking things through with a therapist, are sometimes used for bedwetting. However, research studies that have compared these treatments with more direct approaches (such as the 'buzzer') aimed at increasing bodily controls over the bladder, have demonstrated that the psychotherapy treatments have little effect upon bedwetting. This again indicates that bedwetting is best regarded as nothing more nor less than poor bladder control, and not as some form of emotional disturbance.

Where a child has problems other than bedwetting, or is under more general stresses and anxieties, the doctor or professional adviser may recommend a psychotherapy treatment for these problems – and may sometimes also use a more direct treatment such as drugs or 'buzzer' for the bedwetting. Bedwetting can usually be treated on its own, without ill effects, whether it is the child's only major problem or one of many problems in a child who is also disturbed in various ways.

The enuresis alarm or 'buzzer'. According to the great weight of research that has been conducted into the treatment of bedwetting, the enuresis alarm or 'buzzer' (also sometimes called, rather misleadingly, as it rarely uses a bell, the 'bell-and-pad') has emerged as the most effective. As is often the way of things, it does also demand the greatest effort to produce its results. Although therefore it can produce more, and more long-lasting, cures than drug treatments, it is nothing like as easy to use, and each family considering a choice of treatments must weigh up for themselves the balance between the likely benefits and the costs in terms of effort that each approach involves. In the vast majority of cases the enuresis alarm is likely to be more effective than a psychotherapy treatment, a basic reward system, or simply waiting for a child to grow out of his problem. It is unfortunately true that it is not always easy to find the necessary equipment locally available and with the necessary experienced supervision. Some doctors, health visitors and clinics use the enuresis alarm as their main form of treatment for bedwetting but others have not found it possible to obtain enough equipment or to spend the amount of time necessary to supervise a relatively complex treatment approach conducted by parents and children at home rather than directly by the doctor, health visitor or nurse.

Because of its general effectiveness, and the fact that it is a treatment used at home but is not as simple as it looks, the next two chapters are devoted to the enuresis alarm as a treatment for bedwetting.

4

How 'buzzer' treatment works

The enuresis alarm, 'buzzer' or 'bell-and-pad' is a device used in treating bedwetting to train the body to respond quickly and appropriately to a full bladder during sleep.

The treatment was developed largely by accident. The idea that a device capable of awakening a bedwetting child immediately he had begun to wet might be a useful treatment was put forward as long ago as 1830, but was not reported as having been tried out in practice. Then in 1904, quite independently, a German physician named Pfaundler devised an alarm system for his children's wards in a hospital, with the intention of alerting nurses to wetting incidents when they happened so that beds could be changed and dried without delay. He discovered that for some reason the children's bedwetting reduced as a result. Even then, it was 1938 before Mowrer and Mowrer, the pioneers of the technique, developed it and tried it out, with good results as a treatment method.

The basic idea

The enuresis alarm is designed to produce effective conditions for the learning of night-time bladder control, encouraging this learning where it is not happening under naturally occurring conditions. Whatever the factors that may have led to failure to gain, or the later loss of bladder control, using a special training device and training procedures offers a good chance that the necessary bodily learning will take place. The learning of bladder control through enuresis alarm training does not necessarily follow the same pattern as the normal learning of control during infancy.

An enuresis alarm (see Fig. 7) is simply a device designed to produce a loud sound the moment bedwetting starts to happen at night. A loud sound set off as soon as urine begins to be passed normally produces two reactions. Firstly, the stream of urine is interrupted as the child jumps slightly (the reader may have noticed that normal urination can be

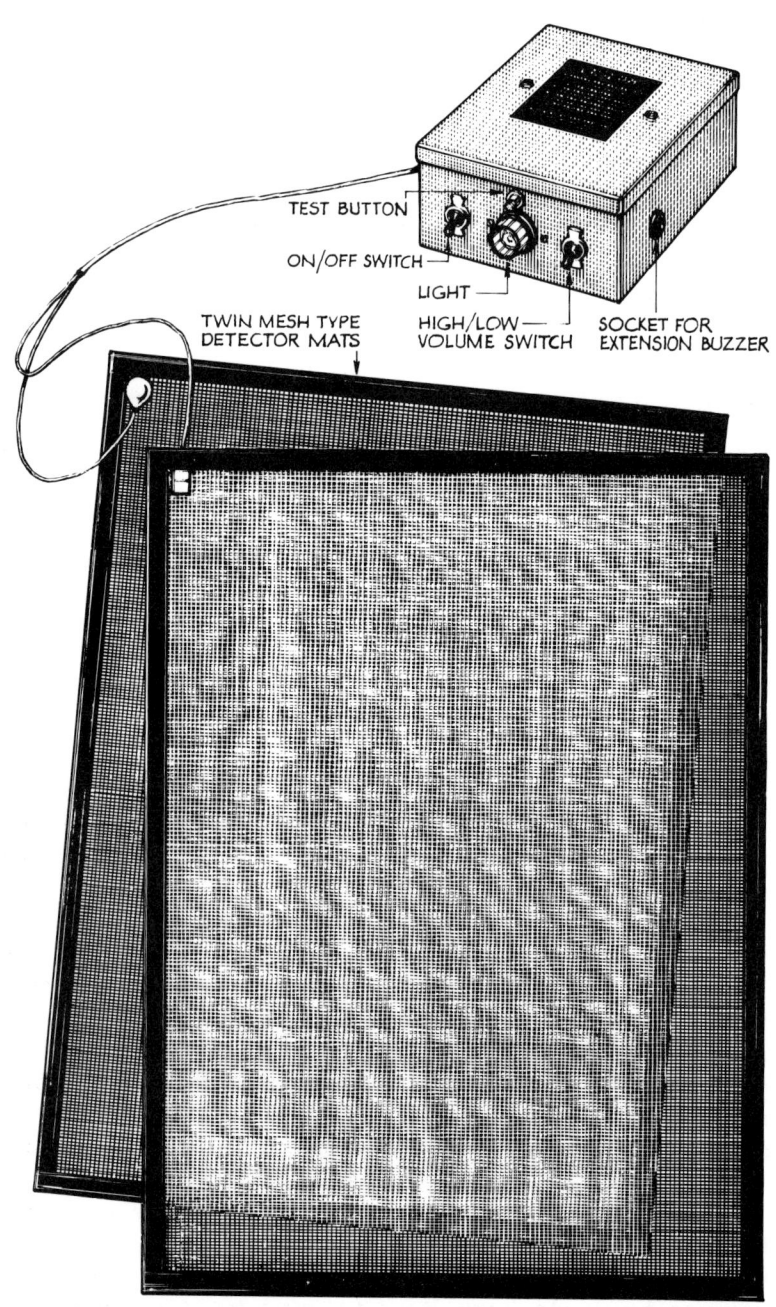

Fig. 7 Typical bedwetting alarm

interrupted if a sudden loud noise occurs). Secondly, the child is woken up by the noise of the alarm.

The alarm device comprises two parts. First, a means of detecting urine as it is passed in the bed, usually by a special detection pad or a pair of simple metal gauze or foil sheets placed in the bed beneath the child. Second, an alarm box containing the sound unit, such as a buzzer or oscillator, plus the necessary battery and circuitry.

The ways in which control is learned

The alarm treatment of bedwetting involves a number of types of learning. The precise blend of learning processes taking place during treatment is likely to differ from one child to another, and may well alter over the length of one course of treatment with any particular child.

A basic type of learning involved in alarm treatment is learning through association (the technical term is 'classical conditioning'). In this way, the bodily reactions of (i) muscular tightening to interrupt or stop the stream of urine, and (ii) waking up, which are produced by the noise of the alarm set off at wetting begins, become associated with the sensation of a full bladder. The process of learning by association is like the one made famous by Pavlov's early experiments in teaching animals to respond to the sound of a bell with the automatic bodily response of producing saliva, by repeatedly associating food with the bell sound. The bedwetting child's association between a full bladder on the one hand, and the 'stopping and waking' produced by the alarm on the other hand, grows in strength as treatment progresses, and his body begins to produce 'stopping and waking' as its own automatic responses to a full bladder, relying less and less on the alarm to make those responses happen. By the end of a successful course of treatment one or both of the stopping and waking responses will begin to occur as the bladder nears its usual 'full' level but well before wetting begins, so that the former bedwetter either holds his urine well enough to last the night without wetting, or wakes in time to visit the toilet. Fig. 8 shows the stages of learning by association through treatment in diagram form. The dotted lines show the links forged by association during treatment.

Because stopping the stream of urine is involved in alarm treatment, first as a reaction to the noise of the alarm and then as a learned response to a full or nearly full bladder, enuresis alarm treatment tends to help a child's ability to hold on to an increased quantity of urine in the bladder. Thus the functional capacity of the bladder will tend to increase. Because

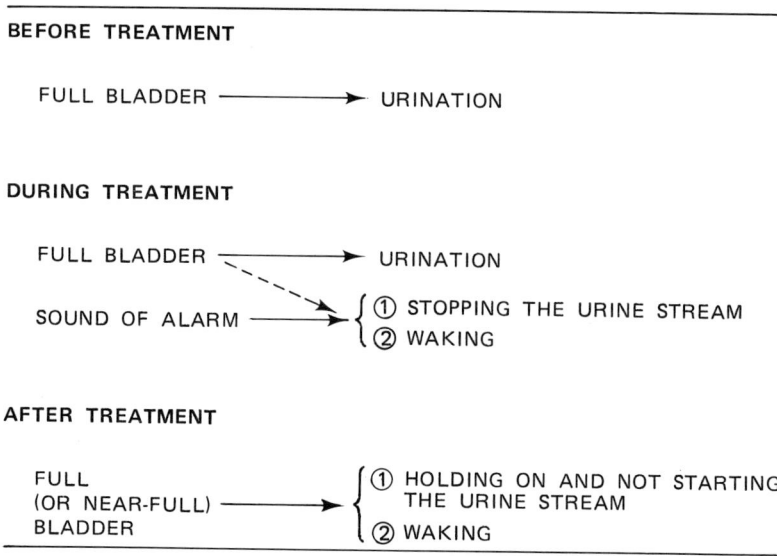

Fig. 8 'Classical' learning in bedwetting alarm treatment

of this, alarm treatment does not always simply train a child to wake up instead of wetting, as is often supposed, but helps some children to hold well enough to store the entire night's output of urine without either wetting or waking. Some children who have been treated with alarms become good 'holders' and so usually sleep the night through, others still need to wake to use the toilet but learn with the alarm to wake well enough and in good time to avoid accidents.

Another type of learning involved in alarm treatment is learning according to the consequences of actions – known technically as 'operant conditioning'. It is known that the strength and probability of repetition of an action may often increase or decrease according to whether the consequences following the action are pleasant or unpleasant. Obviously, rewards and punishments work on this principle, but the ways the body acts and reacts are often moulded or changed by quite subtle, less obvious, and naturally occurring consequences as well.

In alarm treatment, the responses of stopping and waking, first to the alarm sound and then through association to bladder fullness, are strengthened and encouraged because they lead to all the pleasant con-

HOW 'BUZZER' TREATMENT WORKS

sequences of a dry night and to the avoidance of being woken in a wet bed by a noisy alarm. Triggering the alarm by wetting, on the other hand, sets off a sequence of consequences likely to reduce the future probability of wetting – again encouraging the body to perform its new stopping and holding response to achieve this. These include, immediately wetting has begun, a loud noise, disturbed sleep, the discomfort and disappointment of realizing the bed is wet, a trip from bed to the toilet, and the changing of wet sheets. These consequences, occurring immediately wetting begins and so affecting the actions involved in the act of wetting, are more effective than the very remote consequences of waking in a wet bed in the morning without an alarm. Parents who punish a bedwetter when they find the bed wet will have little or no effect at all on the bedwetting (apart from making the child miserable), because this kind of consequence is too remote from the bodily actions that take place at the time of wetting. Only a device like the alarm can act quickly enough to produce consequences likely to affect wetting.

Once the two desired responses of stopping and waking have been learned by association from the alarm, becoming alternatives to wetting when the bladder is full, a full bladder becomes not only the trigger for these two actions but also a signal to the body that selection of the 'stopping and holding' chain of events will lead to more pleasant consequences than selection of the 'automatic wetting' chain of events. There is a great deal of evidence that many of the human body's courses of action are chosen in response to this kind of learned signal (called technically a 'discriminative stimulus'), which is rather like a signpost signalling the consequences at the end of two alternative routes.

In discussing the effects of consequences upon bodily actions, it must again be stressed that this process does not mean that the child could have exercised voluntary or conscious control over the actions that can be influenced by consequences. Actions can be changed over a period of time by their associations and consequences where voluntary effort alone has no effect.

In addition to the types of learning described, there is evidence that impressive procedures and confidence that cure is on its way do contribute significantly to the success of treatment in some unexplained manner. It is well known that even tablets containing no medication at all very often have an effect nevertheless on medical conditions – an odd phenomenon known as the 'placebo effect'. It seems that a placebo effect adds to the effectiveness of the learning processes involved in alarm treatment – children have even been known to improve with alarms that have broken down, and the likelihood of becoming dry without any actual treatment increases markedly as soon as an appointment to start any form of treatment is arranged.

In summary, successful use of an enuresis alarm produces the responses of stopping urination and of waking, links these to bladder fullness through association, and encourages their performance through their consequences.

The following processes in treatment have been identified:
1. The alarm's production of (a) interruption of urination and (b) waking, these being increasingly associated with a full bladder;
2. The encouragement of these responses as an alternative chain of events to bedwetting, because of the very different consequences of each chain of events;
3. The establishment of a bladder at its usual 'full' capacity as (a) a trigger for these new responses, eventually without the help of the alarm, and (b) a signal that the stopping and/or waking chain of events is the one for the body to select to secure the more pleasant consequences;
4. Increase in holding ability and thus the level at which the bladder begins to produce its 'full' reactions;
5. The unexplained 'placebo effect' of confidence in treatment.

Effectiveness

The very numerous research studies of enuresis alarm treatment in use have reported success rates varying widely between 65% and 100%. Overall one may expect a successful outcome with approximately eight out of ten children, assuming properly conducted and well-supervised treatment.

A number of research studies have shown that alarm treatment does far better in producing dry nights than simply leaving a child to 'grow out of it' (as has been noted, between 13 and 16% of bedwetters do 'grow out' of the problem in any given year.) Studies comparing alarm treatment with other approaches have shown that the training effect of the alarm, triggered as it is at the moment of wetting, is far greater than alarm clocks or other means of waking a child at night which are not linked to the moment of wetting. Comparisons between the enuresis alarm and other treatments for bedwetting described in Chapter 3 have found the alarm to be more effective; it is more effective than the 'talking psychotherapy' type of treatment, and has longer-lasting effects for most children than do the various drug treatments.

In speaking of the effectiveness of any form of treatment, it is important to consider how likely it is that a cure may not last, the child 'relapsing' to wetting again sometime later. This has been noted already as the major drawback with drug treatments for bedwetting. The relapse rate of basic alarm treatment used to be approximately one in three of children cured – fewer relapses than one would expect after drug treatment, but still a disappointingly high number. The 'overlearning' technique described in the next chapter, involving extra drinking towards the end of treatment, reduces the chances of relapse by building a 'safety margin' of extra learning into the cure. By adding overlearning to basic alarm treatment, the chances of relapse can be reduced in most cases to just under 13%. Put another way, almost 9 out of 10 children cured by alarm treatment with overlearning will remain dry. It is therefore recommended that overlearning should be used wherever possible.

Although it is effective, it is nevertheless true that the enuresis alarm is extremely hard work for parents and child alike. It should not be taken on lightly, but only after careful weighing of the pros and cons within the family. Some people do in fact prefer wet beds to alarm treatment – although this view should not be adopted if the bedwetting child himself is distressed by his problem. In special enuresis treatment clinics using the alarm, as many as one in every three who begin the treatment will give up before it is completed. Giving up happens quickly where there are unusual practical problems or where progress is not made – which serves to stress the need to have an experienced adviser on alarm treatment available wherever possible to help supervise and to help with problems as they may arise. The most common cause of parents abandoning alarm treatment is the failure of the alarm to awaken the child where there is no experienced adviser to suggest any of the number of possible ways of overcoming this difficulty.

Can success or failure be predicted?

It would of course be very useful indeed if the outcome of a course of treatment could be predicted at the beginning, and many doctors and others are concerned that the alarm may be more or less effective according to factors such as the child's age, sex, or frequency of bedwetting.

Many researchers have explored the possibility that various factors may affect or predict the outcome of alarm treatment. The present writer has conducted a series of investigations into this possibility. However, it does not seem that there are many factors which will generally predict the result of alarm treatment for a particular child. Taking children from as young as four upwards, the effectiveness of alarm treatment is the same at all ages right through to adulthood, boys and girls have equal chances of success, lifelong and 'secondary' (re-started) wetting respond in a similar way, and once-a-week wetting and every-night wetting respond at a comparable rate. Although the treatment involves learning, the outcome of treatment is not affected by the child's intelligence. Importantly, children who have not responded to alarm or other forms of treatment in the past or who have relapsed to wetting again do no worse with a new course of alarm treatment than those who have never been treated before.

Relapse after treatment is also not predictable. Factors such as age, sex, original wetting frequency, lifelong or 'secondary' type of wetting, intelligence, and even whether relapse has happened after treatment in the past, are all unrelated to the likelihood of a child remaining dry or relapsing after treatment.

In conclusion, it would be true to say that the only issues markedly affecting success or failure, and relapse or continued dryness, are the practicalities of treatment and any stresses there may be in the child's life at the time. Clearly, a course of treatment without sufficient commitment from the family, or which runs into difficulties where no-one with the necessary experience can help, will probably not succeed. Stress is known to damage bladder control, and it can both reduce the chances of treatment success and in some cases trigger renewed wetting by breaking down the all-important learning imparted by the alarm. Apart from these issues, all children entering treatment share an equal 8 out of 10 chance of success, and all children cured by an alarm plus overlearning share an equal risk of slightly over one out of ten that they may wet again and need a second course of treatment.

5
Using the enuresis alarm ('buzzer') at home

Suitability of the treatment

Treatment of bedwetting with the enuresis alarm or 'buzzer' may be regarded as the best choice amongst the available range of treatments (described in Chapter 3), provided that its use is practicable in a given situation and provided enough effort and commitment can be put into it. It can be used with children aged from four upwards, and can also be used effectively with mentally handicapped children. It can be used by adults with a bedwetting problem. Enuresis alarms are not suitable for early toilet training of very young children, where nerve and muscle systems are not sufficiently developed for the learning involved to take effect, and they are not suitable for the treatment of wetting problems in the elderly, where the problem is more one of muscular and other deterioration rather than of lack of skill. The buzzer is only suitable for wetting that occurs on average once a week or more.

Buzzers can be used in many situations where conditions may seem far from ideal. A single bedroom for the child being treated is a helpful luxury but by no means a necessity — the majority of the writer's patients have been treated in shared bedrooms, and some have been quite successfully treated in dormitories. As discussed in the previous chapter, alarm treatment is suitable for both boys and girls, even where the same or other forms of treatment have not succeeded in the past. Past failures the writer has encountered at special clinics have often been due to the lack of someone experienced to turn to when the almost inevitable 'hitches' needed to be dealt with.

Medical contact

Parents should always seek a doctor's opinion concerning persistent bedwetting, in case an infection needs attention and to check on the possibility that their child may be one of the very few bedwetters with some other but connected physical problem.

Many doctors and clinics have access to enuresis alarms that can be used in cases they consider suitable, in which case this chapter should help by supplementing the information and supervision available from doctor, health visitor or nurse. Naturally, medical opinion on the alarm and other bedwetting treatments varies, and some doctors and clinics prefer other approaches to the problem. In this case, it is important that parents should discuss the position with their doctor and follow his advice with regard to their particular child. The enuresis alarm is a useful treatment for most children, but your doctor is in the best position to judge whether or not this holds true for a particular boy or girl in their medical care.

In most cases in which a doctor is consulted about a child's bedwetting, he will wish to take a urine specimen to check whether the urine is normal or whether there is evidence of infection or anything else needing attention. Often he will ask for a 'midstream' specimen of urine (an 'MSU'), which simply means, as its name implies, the middle rather than the first part of the urine passed. The reason for this is that the first urine to emerge washes out some skin cells and other matter, and therefore gives a less clear picture than the rest of the contents of the bladder. Taking a urine specimen usually means no more than filling a small bottle for the doctor to send off for testing at the laboratory.

Doctors checking a bedwetting child rarely need to do more than a brief physical examination and take a urine specimen. More complicated checks done at the hospital are usually only arranged where there is good reason to suspect that the problem is more than the straightforward lack of bladder control skills that bedwetting represents in the vast majority of cases.

Types of apparatus

Figure 7 (p.34) illustrates a typical enuresis alarm made up of a buzzer box (containing buzzer, battery and circuitry) and a pair of urine detector mats, connected to the box by a thin cable. A wide variety of alarms is available, and many manufacturers will sell or hire their equipment directly to the public. This may be a way of obtaining a set if none are available locally from doctor or clinic. Apparatus obtained in this way should however only be ordered when one's doctor is in agreement, and provided that he approves the particular type of equipment to be bought, as not all equipment is equally safe. Home-made equipment should not be used. Parents purchasing their own equipment will also need to be sure that their doctor or other responsible professional person is willing to supervise and advise as will almost inevitably become necessary at some point.

Different sounds are produced by different types of alarm, and there can be quite marked differences in sound even between alarms of the same type. The noisiest alarms are not necessarily the most effective at arousing the bedwetting child – children seem to respond to the alarm which is 'right' for them, rather than simply to the one which is loudest. Also, the sound actually reaching the child's ears at night is much affected by the size and furnishing of the bedroom. Extremely loud alarms do produce a somewhat better response, particularly in children making only slow response with treatment, but can be much more disruptive to use. Common battery-powered alarms produce a sound in the region of 80 to 90 decibels. Some alarm boxes allow for a choice or adjustment of the alarm sound produced. If such a facility is incorporated, it is worth experimenting with each sound for one to two weeks at a time to discover whether there is one that is more effective for a particular child.

Some alarms have as an optional extra a plug-in booster-buzzer or vibrator unit. These can be very useful where a child does not respond to a standard alarm, and a unit which emits a low vibrating sound can be particularly effective when placed under the pillow or on the bed-head. An extension buzzer to reach a distant parents' bedroom is also a possibility where parents need to help the child but do not hear the alarm in the child's room. Where this is not available but would be helpful, a standard type of 'baby intercom' between child's and parents' bedroom will serve the same purpose. Many alarm units incorporate a small light, which serves the dual purposes of illuminating the control switch and helping to waken the child. Most children are happier if an alarm waking them also gives some light, so that they are not awoken in a completely dark room. Vibrators and special light units have been used to treat deaf children quite successfully, although this usually requires special (but nevertheless still fairly simple) alarm sets.

Most alarms are battery operated and should never be connected to the mains. Mains-powered equipment is not necessary, and should only be used on professional medical or similar advice and for a good reason.

There are a number of different urine-detection systems currently available. All these devices basically comprise a pair of electrical contacts (electrodes) which trigger the alarm in the alarm box when they are bridged by urine. In some systems, urine simply serves to connect one electrode to the other, closing an electrical circuit so that a current can flow. Urine thus performs the same task as a simple switch would do in the circuit. Other systems use the fact that the combination of certain metals and urine can itself act like a tiny battery, generating its own extremely weak current which is detected by transistorized circuitry in the alarm box. The two electrodes in this system generate a small amount of electricity when soaked in urine but not touching each other.

The design of a urine detector system is critical, since poorly designed (or improperly used) equipment can irritate or damage a child's skin — this, although painless, is unsightly and quite avoidable. Skin damage can occur where it is possible for a current, however small, to flow between electrodes that are touching the child's skin. Such a current, not enough to feel, can run even through the perspiration on the surface of the skin. For this reason to use equipment which simply has two electrodes attached in strips or a coil-pattern on the surface of a rubber or plastic sheet would be unwise, and most types of equipment are designed to avoid both electrodes touching the child's skin simultaneously. Three electrode arrangements, illustrated in Fig. 9, are commonly found. The basic type, and the oldest, has electrodes in the form of a pair of supple metal gauze sheets which are placed one above the other in a 'sandwich', separated by a bed sheet (Fig. 9(A)). It is extremely unlikely in this arrangement that a child will come into contact with two electrodes at once. Figure 9(B) illustrates a variant of this principle, in which instead of being gauze sheets, the top electrode is a metal foil perforated with holes, and the bottom electrode is a plain metal foil sheet. The two detector mats illustrated in Figs. 9(C) and (D) are modern easy-clean systems (easily used as they involve one mat rather than two mats with a separating sheet) in which both electrodes are bonded as metal strips into a rubber or PVC mat. Contact between the child and the electrodes is avoided by recessing the electrode strips some way into the mat and thus below the surface above which the child lies.

The equipment the writer uses with patients at his own clinics is of the older, but still very satisfactory, twin gauze sheet type illustrated in Fig. 9(A). I have not come across any cases of skin damage with this type of detector system.*

One advantage of the 'electricity generating' rather than 'circuit clos-

---

* The writer's clinics are equipped with 'Eastleigh MoH' apparatus, manufactured by N. H. Eastwood and Son Ltd., 70 Nursery Road, London N14 5QH.

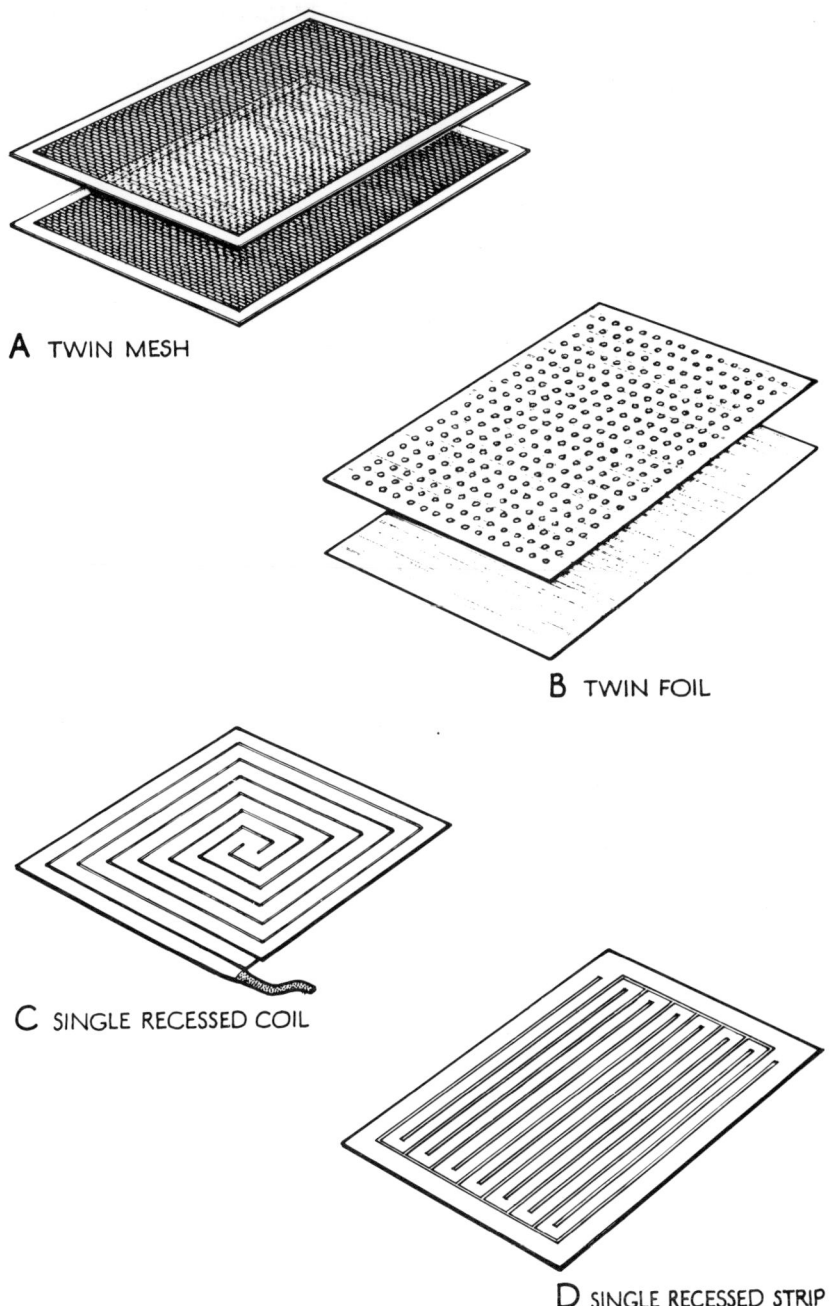

Fig. 9 Different types of urine detector mat

ing' type of detector system is that the former does not have any electrical potential, even from a 6 or 9 volt battery, connected to electrodes in the bed, which reduces the risk of skin damage even further.

There is one further type of detector system that readers may come across, although more commonly used in alarm systems designed for daytime rather than night-time use. This is the system where the electrodes are sewn into a special pad which is either worn in the front and crutch of the child's underpants, or is held in place against the child's body by a simple harness. The system is quite efficient and does not need to be uncomfortable, but does not have any particular advantage over the conventional bed-mat system in treating bedwetting.

Setting up the progress record

At least two weeks (and preferably four weeks) before alarm treatment is begun, it is useful to stop any other special procedures being followed to relieve bedwetting (consulting with the doctor over any procedures or other treatments he has prescribed), and to start keeping a simple record of wet and dry nights. By doing this, a 'baseline' record of the child's own (unaided) bladder control can be obtained, against which progress on the alarm can later be measured. Figure 10 illustrates a simple record chart appropriate for this purpose. The chart for some children will simply show every night wet — but for many the wetting pattern will be very irregular. An irregular wetting pattern is quite normal, and one should avoid the temptation to look for reasons to explain why one night was wet and another dry. With any poorly developed skill, including poor bladder control, successes and accidents will tend to be mixed together more or less at random. The bedwetter will wet frequently and unpredictably for no special reason other than the fact that he is not yet very good at bladder control, just as the toddler learning to walk will frequently fall down for no reason other than the fact that he is not yet very skilful at walking. In both cases, an appropriate record chart would show a thinner scattering of 'accidents' as skill improves.

In a very few cases indeed, there may be some real pattern to wetting, which is likely to show up on a chart kept over a longer time and thus continuing into the treatment period. Some patterns are fairly common and mean little — many children's wetting is slightly worse in colder weather or if they are unwell or anxious about something. Some vary between school and holiday periods — which may be nothing more than the common variation in wetting under different circumstances, and

NIGHT RECORD SHEET

Please check whether the bed is wet or dry each morning. Put 'W' if wet, 'D' if dry.

	WEEK 1	WEEK 2	WEEK 3	WEEK 4	WEEK 5	WEEK 6	WEEK 7	WEEK 8	WEEK 9	WEEK 10	WEEK 11	WEEK 12
MONDAY												
TUESDAY												
WEDNESDAY												
THURSDAY												
FRIDAY												
SATURDAY												
SUNDAY												

Fig. 10 Simple wet/dry chart

may not mean that anything is wrong either at school or at home. A clear pattern, particularly one persisting into treatment, does however suggest a check to see whether there is some source of stress the child would be better without — but it commonly has no significance at all.

Wetting frequencies shown on record charts often differ markedly from one's general estimate of wetting frequencies, and the baseline record is thus particularly useful to ensure that accurate checks on progress can be made later. Because of the usually random pattern of wetting, it is helpful to work out a 'score' of wet and dry nights out of 7 each week, and to plot the weekly score on a graph (as illustrated in Fig. 15, p.58). The randomness of wetting (even during treatment, where more 'D's will begin to be scored) will still cause the weekly scores and thus the graph to vary up and down quite markedly for many children, but the overall level and trend in wetting can usually be seen clearly.

It is useful for the child himself to help to keep his record chart, or take charge of it if old enough. It is not unknown for a child involved in recording his own wetting to improve markedly even before treatment begins. At one clinic of the writer's, almost one in ten children became dry in this way alone.

If the child has other problems of bladder or bowel control, it is useful for some simple record of these to be kept also. Another chart can be used if day wetting is a problem, simply to record days on which it occurred — the purpose is to note whether, as often happens, daytime problems reduce to some extent in line with night wetting. Any urgency or high frequency of urination by day can be rated weekly as 'high', 'moderate' or 'low' and noted to form a record. Reductions in day wetting, urgency or frequency, where present, can be useful early signs that a treatment is having an effect on bladder control.

It is important that the 'W' and 'D' record chart is kept going throughout alarm treatment. It is the only way progress can be monitored. It encourages the child if progress is shown, and highlights the need to review treatment procedures and perhaps seek advice if it is not. Parent and child estimates of changes in wetting during treatment are often quite at variance with the actual situation as shown on an objective record — at special clinics, the writer has often come across families where gradual improvements have gone completely unnoticed until the records are checked, and worse, families convinced that all is well whose records nevertheless show long periods of no improvement that indicate the need to review procedures. Continuation of the simple 'W' or 'D' record illustrated in Fig. 10, with weekly totals added up and perhaps plotted on

NIGHT RECORD

Name ....

Record Commencing ....

Please fill this record in every morning

Morning			Fill in these details if the alarm went off		
	Was the bed Wet (put 'W') or Dry (put 'D')	Did the child wake on his own (without being woken) to use the toilet?	What time (or times) of night did the alarm go off?	Did the alarm wake the child without anyone else helping?	Size of wet patch - put 'S' for small 'M' for medium 'L' for large	Did the child have 'more to do' in the toilet? Put 'S' for small amount 'M' for medium amount 'L' for large amount
Saturday						
Sunday						
Monday						
Tuesday						
Wednesday						
Thursday						
Friday						
Saturday						
Sunday						
Monday						
Tuesday						
Wednesday						
Thursday						
Friday						

Fig. 11 Detailed treatment record chart

a graph at intervals, is all that is necessary. For a younger child, there is no harm, and the possibility of useful encouragement, in turning the chart into a 'star chart' on which the child can stick stars for dry nights (see Fig. 6). If desired, every so many stars can earn a *small* prize or celebration while treatment is in progress.

If parent and child wish to spot early signs of progress, or treatment is not progressing well and the situation needs to be reviewed to highlight problems and monitor the effectiveness of measures to put them right, then the more detailed record chart illustrated in Fig. 11 should be kept. Its use in checking progress or reviewing procedures is described in more detail in later sections of this chapter.

Practical considerations before treatment

Stresses

It is worth considering for a moment before embarking on alarm treatment whether the child is under any emotional stresses that could be relieved. If so, they could hinder the learning processes of treatment if not dealt with, and he will be better off without them anyway. Wetting can be set off after a period of normal bladder control by some stressful situation or event, and although in most cases any stress will have passed and even been completely forgotten, it is just possible that there may be some continuing stress. If nothing springs to mind, no deeper hunting is necessary — and indeed, many cases of 'secondary' wetting are triggered by some change in circumstances which is not necessarily stressful, and others simply occur through no reason other than shaky development of bladder control in the first place.

Where a known stress cannot be relieved — perhaps there are family difficulties or continuing problems at school — alarm treatment can still be used effectively, but as it will have one more obstacle to overcome it will need more care, patience and probably persistence than where everything else is going well. There is no reason why alarm treatment should not be used where the child has other psychological problems — these often do not even hinder progress, and if the bedwetting is successfully relieved, other problems are unlikely to be affected positively or negatively, and at least the child will end up with one problem less.

Previous experience of treatment

A child's chances of success are not affected by past failures at alarm treatment, or in cases where he has 'relapsed' to wetting again after an initial success. Any problem met with in the course of previous treatment should however be noted and a solution worked out or advice sought before trying again. This chapter may suggest some solutions.

Sleeping arrangements

Two thirds of the children treated by the writer with alarms have used them in shared bedrooms. The usual pattern is that when the alarm is first used, others are awoken by it — but they soon become used to it and often stir little or not at all. The change is rather like sleeping in a room near a noisy railway — at first, one is disturbed a great deal by the sound, but eventually one adjusts to it and hardly notices it. The alarm-user, and the parent who helps him at night, do not make this adjustment as they respond to each alarm triggering with a definite routine.

Shared bedrooms can be a positive asset where a child has difficulty in waking to the alarm, as a brother or sister can often help.

Many people using an alarm in the family are concerned at the possibility of the noise disturbing neighbours; while this is not impossible, it is amazing how much sound is absorbed by walls. A more common problem is the parent in another bedroom in the same house failing to hear the alarm!

Bedding

Using an alarm with the basic sandwich detector mat system requires one extra layer of bed-linen; a sheet, drawsheet or pillowcase. The bed will also need changing after each wetting at night. Until treatment begins to have an effect, therefore, some additional bedding and some extra washing (though not necessarily much more than usual) will be needed.

It is important that the sheets used in setting up a bed containing an alarm detector mat should not be made of nylon, even though it is easy to wash. Nylon tends to encourage perspiration, which causes problems by triggering the buzzer on an otherwise dry bed, and it does not allow urine to pass through to the detector electrodes quickly enough to enable the necessary rapid detection of the start of wetting.

More than one bedwetter

Where more than one child wets the bed in the family, only one at a time should be treated with an alarm. Two alarms in the same house can cause chaos! The choice as to who should be first is for the family to make together, but preference may perhaps be given to the child most distressed about wetting, the most frequent bedwetter or, these factors being equal, the oldest child.

Explaining to the child

It is extremely important that the child should have the problem of bedwetting, the use of the alarm, and the way it is to go about teaching his body what to do to stay dry, explained carefully and in terms he can understand. The alarm can seem a frightening piece of equipment, and reassurance is needed that its wires will not be attached to the child himself, that he will not have an electric shock, and that the whole thing is basically simple and friendly. A negligible proportion of children are frightened by the alarm if properly acquainted with it in the first place. Older children appreciate a sensible explanation of the principles and procedures involved.

In explaining bedwetting to a child, it is helpful to point out that all children find their bodies are good at some things and poor at others. Some are good footballers or swimmers, others are not very good at these things. In just the same way, some are good at controlling their bladders, others not very good. Children who find bladder control a problem are not odd or peculiar, any more than children who are no good at football or cannot swim are odd or peculiar. Being not very good at controlling one's bladder is just as common as being no good at some sport or another. In either case, special coaching can improve matters, and this is where the buzzer comes in.

The way the buzzer helps can be explained to a child along the lines of the following, according to age:

> 'When you have a wet night, what happens is that the tank inside you, called your bladder, gets full and sends a message to your brain saying that it needs to be emptied. Your brain, though, is too sleepy to take any notice, so your bladder just has to empty in your bed and you have a wet night. When you are using the alarm, the buzzer wakes you up and stops you wetting as soon as this happens.

USING THE ENURESIS ALARM ('BUZZER') AT HOME

After a while, your brain gets so used to being woken up just after it gets that message saying that your bladder is full, that instead of staying sleepy it learns to listen to what your bladder is saying, and either wakes you up in time to go to the toilet or tells you to hold on for a while.'

Setting up the apparatus

Different types of equipment need slightly different procedures, but the principles are similar. This section describes the setting up of alarms

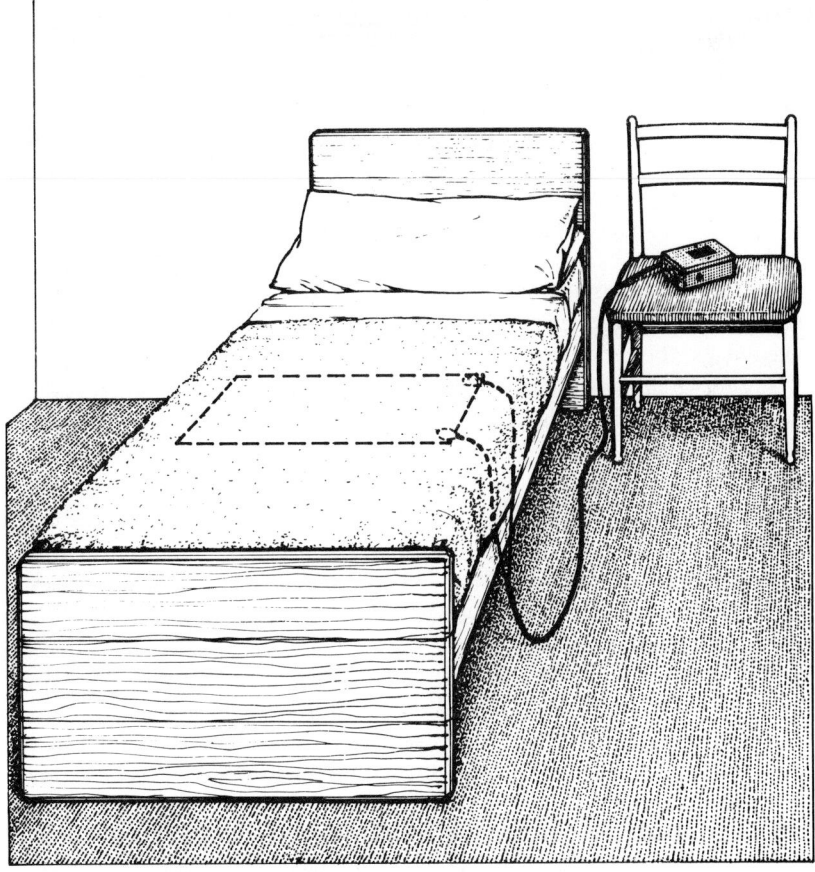

Fig. 12 Detector mats across the bed. Cable positioned to avoid child tripping over it

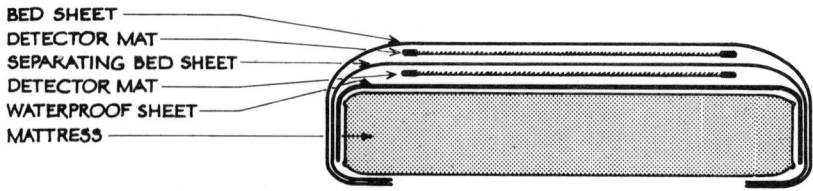

Fig. 13 Section of twin mat arrangement in the bed

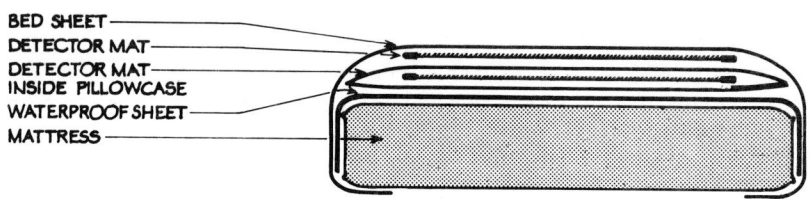

Fig. 14 . . . using pillowcase

using twin wire mesh sheets as a urine detector system. For other equipment, the maker's instructions will give any other information needed for their particular set.

Figure 12 shows the correct positioning of the detector mats across the part of the bed where the child wets. It is in fact rare for a child to 'miss' the detector mats or pad. Figure 13 shows the 'sandwich' arrangement of the mats in cross-section as they should be positioned, one above the other, beneath the child. The layers, starting from the mattress at the bottom, are:

1. Waterproof sheet (suitable sheets can be obtained from most baby shops, or a small camping-type groundsheet with eyelets for easy tying can be used).
2. First wire detector mat. With alarms using mats of two different colours (the different metals used in the 'generating' rather than 'bridging the gap' electrode system), it does not matter which goes on the bed first. With foil sheets, the one without holes goes on first.
3. Separating bed sheet (not made of nylon). This is to keep the mats above and below from actually touching each other. If they do touch, alarms using the 'bridging the gap' detector system will immediately go off, while those using the 'generating' principle

will not work even if the child wets. To perform its task, the separating sheet should not be torn or threadbare, but it need not cover the whole bed as long as it is big enough to keep the mats apart with a tuck at the sides and good 'border' around the mats. A half-sheet or cot-sheet will do. An alternative is to place the lower detector mat *inside* a pillowcase (not nylon), thus dispensing with the need for a separating sheet. This arrangement is illustrated in Fig. 14.

4   Second wire detector mat, positioned on top of the separating sheet, directly above the lower mat. The connecting terminal needs to be on the same side of the bed as that of the first mat, and for the sake of comfort the two terminals should not be directly on top of one another (this can be avoided by turning one the other way up).

5   Bed sheet (again, not nylon). This covers the mat arrangement, and is the bottom sheet on which the child lies. Although aware of the detector pads beneath them, children do not usually find them particularly uncomfortable.

The leads to the bedside alarm box should be connected to the mats according to the manufacturer's instructions; most alarms use some form of snap connector. If possible, the leads may be left permanently clipped to the mats to avoid wear and tear on the connectors, which are relatively weak points in the detector mats. The alarm box should be placed on a table or chair, or on the floor by the child's bed — positioned so that he will not trip over the lead, and put far enough away to require him to rise from the bed to switch it off.

It is helpful if the bed is made up with the alarm well before bedtime on the first night of treatment. If one can spare the sheets, any fears a child may have (or the curiosity of an older child as to how it all works) can be met by a practice triggering of the buzzer. To do this, set up and switch on the alarm, then pour a small quantity of water with some salt dissolved in it onto the detector mat 'sandwich'. (Although many alarms will trigger with fresh water, some need salty water.) Firm hand pressure should then be put onto the wet patch for a few seconds until the buzzer triggers, to ensure good contact through the detector 'sandwich' as the child's own weight does in normal use.

As well as demonstrating the alarm in this way, parents should encourage a young or nervous child to play with the buzzer until it is familiar and no longer a frightening object. Misuse or dismantling the buzzer is not exactly to be encouraged, but many children whose response on first seeing their alarm was tearful have happily gone to bed with it after half-an-hour pretending its sound is a police siren. The practice triggering by salt water is useful to test the proper operation of the alarm if some fault is suspected.

Nightly routine

While using the alarm, the child should sleep without wearing anything below the waist. The reason for this is that pyjama trousers, underpants or long nightdresses tend to soak up some of the urine before it can reach the detector mats, so delaying the sounding of the buzzer. This sort of delay can seriously reduce the effectiveness of treatment.

If a child is too embarrassed to sleep naked below the waist, even with a dressing-gown ready to grab before leaving the bed, *thin* pyjama trousers or pants (not nylon) may be tried as a last resort – but not if there are problems in waking to the alarm, and accepting that response to treatment may be slowed down.

Older girls are often worried about using the alarm while they are having a period. A tampon however will not affect urine detection in any way; if by chance blood does reach the detector mats all that will happen is a 'false alarm' triggering of the buzzer.

When the alarm goes off at night, the child must:
1   switch the buzzer off as quickly as he can;
2   visit the toilet to finish emptying his bladder there, or use a pot in the bedroom;
3   help his parent to remake the bed with dry sheets and dried detector mats;
4   switch the alarm back on;
5   return to bed.

Parents need to do the following while their child is using the alarm:
1   Make sure the alarm is in use and switched on every night. It should be used every night except for very occasional special reasons – if the child is ill, if there are visitors sleeping in the house, or if the child is sleeping away from home.
2   Avoid:
    (a)   'lifting' – i.e. waking the child to visit the toilet when the alarm has not gone off;
    (b)   restricting fluids; a child on the alarm should be allowed a

USING THE ENURESIS ALARM ('BUZZER') AT HOME

drink whenever he is thirsty, even last thing at night.

3   When the alarm goes off at night, help the child to wake, and guide him if necessary to switch the alarm off and visit the toilet or pot. (A child who is afraid of the dark should not be left to go to the toilet alone.) Where (as often happens) the alarm has not woken the child by the time a parent gets there, *immediately* waken the child *while the alarm continues to sound*, encouraging him to switch off *himself*, but guiding his hand if necessary, and only switching off for him if he really is too unaware of events to do so. Parents should not switch the alarm off before waking the child, as this prevents the important association between the alarm sound and waking.

4   Once the child has gone to the toilet or pot to 'finish off', remake the bed with dry bedclothing. Wipe the detector mats dry, with a dry corner of the sheet being taken off, and set the alarm up again in case of a second wetting. Depending upon age and how awake he is, the child can help – older children who wake well to the alarm can cope completely on their own.

If bedclothes are in short supply or the disturbance is proving too much, the bed can be remade without the alarm until the next night, so that there is never more than one buzzer call in any one night. Many children only wet once in a night in any case. Those that wet more than once are helped more if none of the wets are 'missed', but usually carry on progressing even with only the first wet each night 'caught' by the buzzer.

5   In the morning, fill in 'W' for wet or 'D' for dry on the record chart, with the child. Even a small wet patch should be entered as 'W' – for a 'D', the bed must have stayed completely dry all night. If the buzzer gave a 'false alarm' (where this happens, it is usually triggered by perspiration), there will have been no wet patch with clear edges to it, and it should not be counted as a wet bed.

Wet sheets should be washed before re-use, and not simply be dried out over a radiator or elsewhere, even if the wet patch was small, since the dried residue in the sheets will leave the alarm very easily triggered by perspiration, making false alarms more likely. Sheets that have become damp enough with perspiration to trigger the alarm should also be washed before re-use, for the same reason.

Signs of progress

Alarm treatment is a process of learning, and each buzzer triggering may be seen as another lesson in bladder control. Learning any sort of skill is a gradual process, and the alarm is not a 'magic box' that can produce sudden learning or sudden results. Some children do respond quicker than others, but the average length of treatment is three months, and often no change is noticed for the first month. The progress made through this learning, as with other forms of learning, is uneven and often includes setbacks as it progresses.

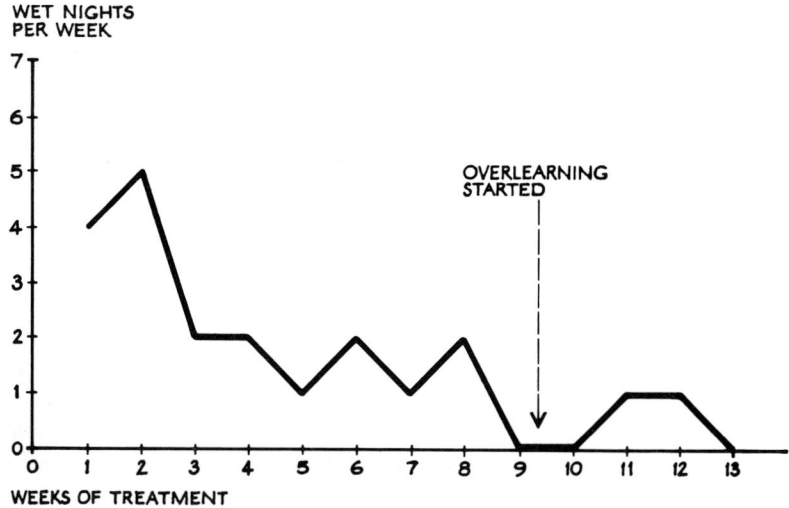

Fig. 15 Typical treatment record graph (actual patient)

Figure 15 shows a typical graph of wet nights per week during alarm treatment. ('Overlearning' is the procedure designed to increase the chances of staying dry for good and described in the next section of this chapter.) The graph shown is the actual record of a child treated by the writer, who remained completely dry after treatment.

The following are the most important signs of progress in alarm treatment (although they do not all occur in all cases, and do not occur in any given order).

More urine to 'finish off' in the toilet

As the child's wetting is 'turned off' more efficiently once the buzzer is triggered, more remains to be emptied when he then reaches the toilet or pot to finish off.

Smaller wet patches

Again, as the child's body learns to shut off the stream of urine more quickly and efficiently, less is emptied into the bed and the wet patch becomes smaller. Usually, the first step is the patch varying in size rather than being always large or the bed being soaked. It then settles to a more steady reduction in size.

Only one wet per night

Those children who wet more than once each night usually reduce to once only after two to three weeks, if it is possible for the alarm to be used to 'catch' every wetting.

Better waking to the alarm

Children often do not wake to the alarm without help at first. Some never wake without help – but are cured by the alarm all the same if help arrives fairly quickly. Improved waking often develops during treatment, shown by the child more frequently 'beating' his parent to the buzzer when it is triggered, and being more aware of what is going on once he has woken.

Reduced daytime problems

As bladder control begins to improve, urgency and frequency of visits to the toilet by day, if high to start with, will improve and any daytime wetting will often reduce. This usually happens before much of an increase in dry nights is noticed. Any daytime wetting is sometimes cured altogether by night-time alarm treatment.

More dry nights

This usually follows other signs of progress, and happens most in the second and third months of an average course of treatment.

Self-waking to visit the toilet

The buzzer teaches the child's body to hold on to urine and/or to wake up to urinate. Some children hold on more as their main response to treatment, others wake more. Waking themselves in good time to visit the toilet to empty the bladder is an important sign of progress for many children.

The end of treatment and overlearning

Alarm treatment as described should be continued until 14 dry nights *in a row* have been achieved. This usually takes some 8 to 12 weeks, although it can happen quickly for some children who might already have been 'almost there'. It does not however take any longer for children whose wetting was more frequent to begin with.

If one stopped using the alarm at the 14 dry nights stage, the chances of renewed wetting in the near future would be around one in three. To reduce this to only a little over one in ten, 'overlearning' should be used, provided there is no medical reason against its use.

Overlearning should be started as soon as the row of 14 dry nights is completed. While continuing to use the alarm as before, the child should now take extra drinks in the last hour before going to bed. He may take as much as he can comfortably manage, and may spread the extra drinking out over the hour and have a variety of different types of drink. Most children manage a pint to a pint and a half – but no more than two pints should be taken and the child should not drink so much that he feels discomfort.

The extra drinking should be repeated each night, while carrying on with the alarm. This overlearning usually causes more wets and thus alarm triggerings (as can be seen in the example in Fig. 15) – but this also means extra 'lessons in control' that build up a safety margin of extra learning to make continued dryness more certain (hence the term *over*-learning). Some children are lucky enough to have gained such strong learning during the earlier part of treatment to remain dry in spite of the extra fluids. One likely effect of overlearning is to increase the functional capacity of the bladder, and thus its holding ability (see Chapter 2).

Nine out of ten children can cope with overlearning and will become dry again on the alarm even while drinking the extra fluids. If however the child returns to over 4 wet nights per week on overlearning, or renewed wetting fails to reduce after two weeks of overlearning, the extra drinking should be abandoned. No fluid restriction should however be introduced instead. Alarm treatment is then continued until a further 14 dry nights in a row are achieved, when treatment may be stopped. Time will have been lost, but to try overlearning is worth it for a nine out of ten chance of a significantly more long lasting cure. A child who cannot cope with overlearning is not especially likely to relapse to wetting – his chance of relapse remains at around one in three after he has regained 14 dries.

Assuming all goes well on overlearning, the alarm and extra fluids at bedtime should be continued until 14 dry nights in a row are again reached, and then the alarm may be removed and extra drinks stopped. The child may then drink when thirsty, without fluid restrictions.

Relapse after treatment

After completing treatment, the occasional wet night as things settle down is quite common and nothing at all to worry about. For the child who does restart regular wetting in the future (which happens in about 13% of children treated with overlearning), this is disappointing but not a disaster, as he will respond to a second course of treatment as well as to the first, and be no more likely to relapse again than any other child being treated for the first time. There are not many children the writer has ever had to treat more than twice. A second course of treatment can be considered if wetting has returned for one or more nights per week on average. This can be checked by restarting a chart – which as has been noted can help to reduce problems even by itself.

At the end of a successful course of treatment all children have a nearly nine out of ten chance of remaining dry without needing any further treatment or special effort. Relapses can happen simply because bladder control always has been a difficult skill for children who have been bedwetters, or can be triggered by something stressful or by a straightforward and non-stressful change of circumstances. They mean nothing more than that some children need two sessions rather than one of training in bladder control before the skill is secure. Refresher courses are a part of learning many kinds of skill.

Problems and solutions

Most courses of treatment run into problems at some stage, and success depends upon their quick solution. This section describes some of the most common problems, and basic ways of dealing with them. If treatment starts to run into difficulties, the detailed record chart illustrated in Fig. 11 (p.49) should be kept instead of the simple 'W' and 'D' chart; it will identify problems such as non-waking, failure of the stream of urine to be 'shut off' by the alarm, and false alarms. It will also monitor the effectiveness of steps taken, as described below, to solve such problems.

Not waking to the alarm

Few children are always woken to the buzzer without the help of a parent, brother or sister at the start of treatment. Most, however, will wake much better as time goes on, provided parents stick to the procedure of never turning the buzzer off before the child has been woken to turn if off himself.

To become dry, a child on alarm treatment must have at least one of the two basic reactions to the buzzer sound — that is, shutting off the stream of urine, and waking. Most children have both, but it is quite common for a child with one but never the other to be successfully cured. Thus the boy or girl who never wakes without help will probably succeed *provided* the buzzer causes him to stop in midstream. This will be happening satisfactorily if the child has more to do on reaching the toilet after a buzzer triggering and if his patch sizes in the bed are becoming smaller. Both these signs will be recorded on the detailed record chart. If these signs are present, it is enough to continue simply waking the child as soon as his buzzer goes — helping him to wake, then helping him in turning the buzzer off, and always going quickly to him rather than waiting to see if he will wake on his own. Any progress in self-waking will appear on the detailed chart where a record is kept of how often the child beats his parent to the off-switch.

Some children are still very confused and sleepy even when woken by a parent after a buzzer triggering. They need physical guidance to switch the buzzer off and visit the toilet — and some have been known to begin getting ready for school, or worse to try using a non-existent toilet unless guided to the real one! Guidance is needed, but the buzzer will not harm such a child.

If difficulty in waking is a problem, any of the following that are feasible may be attempted to improve the situation, while monitoring on the detailed chart. It must be remembered that apart from extremely loud buzzers, it is the *right* sound rather than the *loudest* sound that is being sought.

1   Adjust the alarm sound if the set in use has this facility.
2   Exchange buzzers – even two buzzers of the same type will give very different sounds.
3   Place the buzzer box inside an open biscuit tin.
4   Renew the battery in the alarm to improve the sound.
5   Use a plug-in booster buzzer or vibrator (attached perhaps to the bedhead or placed under the pillow) if obtainable.
6   Check that procedures are being followed properly – particularly that no pyjama trousers, underpants or long nightdresses are being worn.

If non-waking persists but there are other signs of progress, there is little cause for concern. If, however, there are no other signs of progress, and particularly if there is no more to do on reaching the toilet, or parents do not hear the buzzer, some children can be trained to wake to the buzzer by being woken to its sound for two or three randomly-spaced times each night (between their bedtime and that of their parents). The parent should trigger the buzzer sound using the test-button usually provided, waking the child up while the buzzer sounds. The child may then switch the buzzer off, visiting the toilet if he wants to. The alarm should be left in use to catch wettings as usual. This routine may be tried for two or three weeks and its effects on waking to a 'real' buzzer triggering monitored on the detailed chart.

Not 'shutting off' the stream of urine

The reaction of shutting off the stream of urine to the sound of the buzzer is the other central 'building brick' of alarm treatment. Its occurrence can be monitored by recording on the detailed chart the wet patch size, and whether there is more to do on reaching the toilet. If progress is slow and the detailed chart shows that this reaction is not occurring, the steps just described to help with non-waking should be tried to help the stimulus of the buzzer sound to get through.

If these do not have an effect on the recorded signs of 'shutting off', the following special training routine can be tried – and monitored – over a period of two to three weeks. On at least one visit the child makes to the toilet to empty his bladder each day while at home (probably in the evening), he should be accompanied by a parent (or brother or sister) carrying the alarm box. In order to link 'shutting off' with the buzzer sound, and to increase the likelihood of the child's body recalling the link at night, the buzzer should be set off (again by the test button or by short-circuiting the mats, depending on alarm type) as soon as he has started the urine stream. The child should then try to 'shut off' – he will quite probably not succeed at first. If he succeeds, the buzzer should be turned off and urination then completed – with congratulations on a task achieved!

Damaged or worn detector mats

One set of detector mats is not always enough to last a complete course of treatment, although the durability of different designs of mat varies. Damaged or worn mats should be replaced; broken wires can disrupt treatment by producing false alarms or by putting the buzzer temporarily out of action through a short-circuit between sandwich-type mats, and can be uncomfortable and scratchy. As a temporary measure a scratchy break in wires can be covered by a piece of waterproof sticking plaster.

False alarms

Buzzers do sometimes trigger on a bed that has not been wet, and in some courses of treatment such false alarms can become a major problem. False alarms do not count as a wet bed on the record chart. It is very common for children not to be woken by a false alarm, even if they normally wake well to the buzzer, because the alarm sound is not linked in a false alarm to the stimulation of a full bladder. A child woken by a false alarm need not visit the toilet if he does not want to.

The usual cause of false alarms is dampening of the bed-sheets by perspiration, although any other body fluid (such as blood or saliva) will set the buzzer off. Faulty or over-sensitive equipment is a less common but possible cause. The following are the steps to take.

1   Check detector mat or mats for short circuits because of broken wires poking through the separating sheet of 'sandwich' types, or because of a hole or a threadbare sheet. Solve respectively by covering the broken wire with a sticking plaster until mats can be replaced, or by replacing the separating sheet. Put the lower mat inside a pillowcase if the child's movement at night causes the mats to touch.
2   Reduce the tendency to perspire by reducing the quantity of bedclothing and the bedroom temperature, if excessive. Avoid

waterproof-encased mattresses, which can be hotter to sleep on than a normal mattress covered with a single waterproof sheet.
3   Remove bottom sheet and separating sheet after a false alarm; their re-use while damp with perspiration can lead to further false alarms. The removed sheets should be washed to remove salty deposits before re-use, to reduce the risk of repeated false alarms.
4   Reduce alarm sensitivity and absorb more of the perspiration by doubling or even tripling the separating sheet between sandwich-type detector mats, or the cover sheet over single-pad detector mats. The child may for the same purpose be allowed to wear pyjama trousers (in preference to underpants, as the latter cover less and are thus less efficient), of a material other than nylon.

Alarm failure

If the alarm does not work when the bed is wet, it may be tested quickly by means of the test button provided on most sets, or more thoroughly by a practice triggering using salt water and firm hand pressure on a normally set up bed. The following common causes may be checked and rectified as appropriate if the alarm still fails to sound:
1   Incorrect arrangement of detector mats or incorrect or poor connections from bed to alarm.
2   Run-down battery.
3   A short circuit between detector mats or electrodes, which will silence certain types of alarm while triggering false alarms in others.
4   Damage within the alarm box if it has been dropped or roughly handled.
5   Someone (patient, brother or sister perhaps) turning the buzzer off before settling down for the night is not unknown!

Alarm treatment with the handicapped child

Alarm treatment can be used quite successfully with children having a variety of mental or physical handicaps. In the case of a physical handicap, the doctor should be consulted over the suitability of the alarm. Broadly however, treatment can usually be adapted around a handicap that affects mobility (by counting on parental help to switch the buzzer off and by use of a bottle for urination where the toilet cannot be reached). In the case of a handicap in which the physical aspects of bladder control are affected (as in some forms of paralysis), control may be impossible and the alarm therefore inappropriate. There are some marginal cases however in which a doctor may consider that an alarm may help to make the best use of what ability to control has been left by a partial impairment. As the alarm uses sound to produce its reactions, deafness is an obvious problem, although use of plug-in vibrator units can overcome this problem in some cases, and special equipment using a bright light rather than a loud noise has been found effective.

The alarm is a suitable treatment for mentally handicapped children provided its use is practicable with the particular child. Although the treatment relies on learning, it is such basic body-learning that success

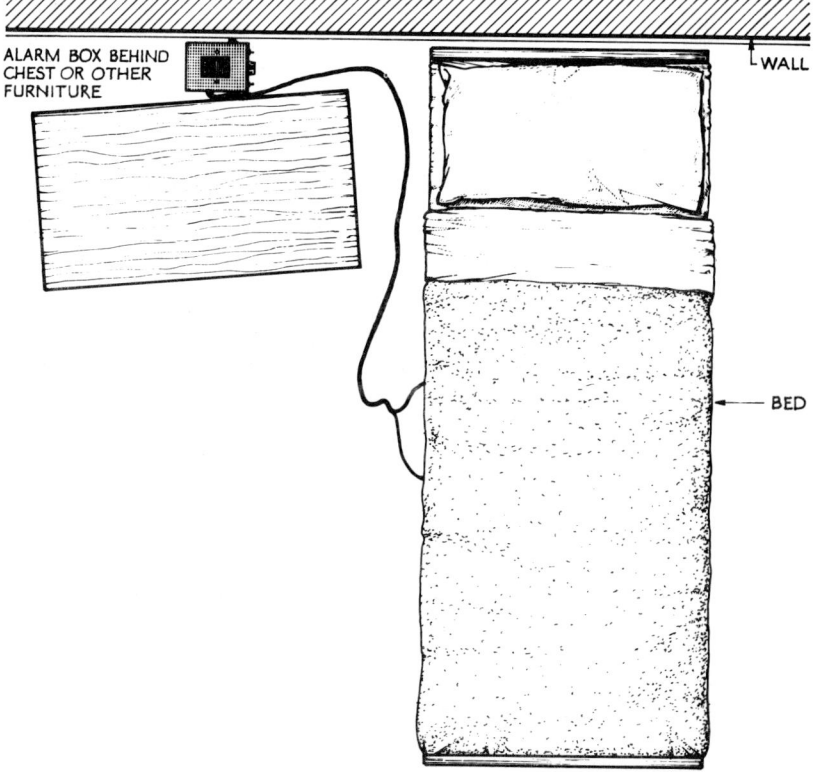

Fig. 16 'Buzzer' box behind furniture (requiring child to rise in order to switch off)

does not require high levels of intelligence, and can be achieved despite a mental handicap.

Special allowances do have to be made in treating a mentally handicapped child, however — particularly because explanation is difficult and the child can often take little active role in his treatment. The buzzer's presence and its sound often need introducing *gradually*, in small doses rather than suddenly. The buzzer can be placed and sounded at a considerable distance from the child at first, while he is happy at something else, and brought closer in stages when he accepts it without fear. It can then be set up in the bedroom. Parents will need to help most mentally handicapped children to wake, switching the buzzer off after waking and guiding to the toilet or pot. Sometimes a child will chew through the alarm lead, and this can often be routed under the bed and taped to avoid tempting lengths of lead. If the alarm box itself is a source of temptation, or is 'hauled in' for attention on the end of its lead, it can often be wedged on the floor behind a piece of furniture angled to the wall (as in Fig. 16).

In treating a mentally handicapped child, one must look out for inappropriate reactions to the alarm, and if necessary abandon the attempt if these cannot be resolved. One fairly common problem of this sort is the child who remains afraid of the alarm despite a gradual introduction. He should not be pushed, or future and possibly more successful attempts might be prejudiced. A second is the child who actually enjoys the buzzer too much and will deliberately urinate when awake to hear it go off! This learning is hardly to be encouraged. If such difficulties occur, the chances of eventual success will be greater if the treatment is postponed and tried afresh in not less than three months' time, when the child's reaction is very likely to be quite different.

6

Daytime pants wetting

Nature and incidence

Daytime pants wetting ('diurnal enuresis') is less common than bedwetting, affecting something between one and three per cent of all school age children. It is usually linked with bedwetting, and is an additional problem for around a quarter of bedwetters. Day wetting without any night-time wetting is relatively uncommon, and unlike bedwetting is to be found more often amongst girls than boys. The likelihood of a child growing out of day wetting is similar to the likelihood of bedwetting disappearing on its own as time passes — about 15 out of every 100 wetters will grow out of the problem within the period of a year, without anything special being done.

Urinary tract infections are rather more likely in children with a day wetting problem, and can be one of its causes. The possibility of an infection should therefore be checked with a doctor, as should the possibility of a physical problem needing further investigation or treatment.

Urgency and frequency

Urgency and frequency in going to the toilet to urinate very commonly accompany daytime wetting. Indeed, in many cases daytime wetting is simply the result of not reaching the toilet in time, when wetting is urgent and too frequent for toilets always to be easily available. The child may receive little or no warning that the bladder needs emptying, and some receive no warning at all until wetting has started.

Two factors are commonly present in daytime wetting, and can result in urgency and frequency. Firstly, the pelvic floor muscles between the child's legs may not be efficient enough to keep the bladder opening raised and so closed, thus there is little resistance before bladder emptying starts. Secondly, the detrusor muscle that makes up the walls of the bladder can be overactive, quick to produce frequent and strong contractions and so to begin bladder emptying.

One other factor is important in urgency and day wetting. As noted in Chapter 2, most people experience increasing urgency as they walk towards the toilet. Moderately urgent urination can become desperate as the toilet is reached. For the child (or adult) with problems in the skills of control, perhaps with an overactive bladder and an inefficient pelvic floor as 'gatekeeper', urgency can rise so quickly and so far that wetting starts well before the toilet is ever reached. For some, starting on the way to the toilet or even thinking of going can prove too much. For others, a steep rise in urgency can cause leakage just as the toilet is reached – 'going earlier' is of course not a solution to this, as it is the act of going towards the toilet that is actually triggering the problem.

Stress incontinence

One form of daytime wetting happens when a physical stress squeezes on the bladder and forces some urine out – this leakage is known as 'stress incontinence'. It can happen during coughing, sneezing, laughing or while straining the body in lifting or stretching. Quite a few children will 'leak' a little if they are tickled, and the expression 'wetting oneself with laughter' refers to the problem. Stress incontinence is common in children with other daytime bladder control difficulties, and is also common in women after childbirth (where the all-important pelvic floor has been damaged), men after a prostate operation (where the pelvic floor has been affected by the surgery) and in the elderly where the muscles of control are losing their efficiency with age.

Figure 2 (p.6) showed how the bladder outlet is closed by the pelvic floor which surrounds the tube (urethra) leading from the bladder to the outside world. Normally, when an action such as coughing squeezes the bladder itself, the same pressure also squeezes against the urethra, just below the bladder, keeping it shut and preventing leakage. If the pressure on the urethra in not enough, leakage and stress incontinence will result.

'Giggle micturition'

Usually in stress incontinence, the leakage of urine stops once the physical stress (such as laughing or coughing) has stopped. Some children, particularly girls, find however that the flow of urine continues until the bladder is emptied. The upward tightening of the pelvic floor to shut off the urine stream is in these cases not strong enough to resist the powerful emptying contractions of the bladder wall muscle, which usually die away in straightforward stress incontinence as the pelvic floor shuts off the flow. This problem bears the impressive name of 'giggle micturition' because it is often triggered by laughing.

Ways of improving the situation

The following sections suggest ways in which parents and children can themselves help to reduce daytime urine control problems. Whichever approach is tried, a record of progress should be kept so that the usefulness of each can be assessed, and used as the basis for a decision to abandon or continue any particular approach after giving it a trial: a reasonable trial period for any of the following would be one month.

Holding practice

One way to help reduce daytime bladder control problems such as urgency, frequency and pants wetting, is to practice the 'holding' of urine before emptying the bladder. Holding practice can increase the functional capacity of the bladder (the amount it can comfortably contain), and as has been seen this is one of the key factors in bladder control. It is not however the only one, and other measures may be needed as well in some cases.

To practice holding, either of two approaches may be adopted. The first is for the child to visit the toilet at regular intervals 'by the clock' — perhaps every hour through the day — and then to lengthen the period between visits in five-minute stages once the previous holding period has been comfortably achieved for a number of consecutive occasions. The lengthening of holding periods may be continued until a natural limit is reached beyond which progress is no longer made, or until the child can hold comfortably between five or six urinations a day. Holding practice need not be continued further than this, and should not be continued in any case if there is discomfort.

The second approach is to practice holding for a short period once the first urge to empty the bladder is felt and before going to the toilet, provided the problems are minor enough for this to be achieved without accidents. The first stage is to count ten seconds before leaving for the toilet, progressing when this is comfortably achieved to counting twenty seconds, waiting half a minute, a full minute, then a minute and a half, continuing in half-minute steps until ten minutes can comfortably be managed. Again, this length of time need not be exceeded, and holding practice should be discontinued if there is any discomfort.

Holding practice, by either approach, is best tried during school holidays, as it is far more difficult — and is not always possible at all — at

Name .... Record commencing ....

Fill the date each morning, and then fill in a new line each time you <u>either</u> visit the toilet <u>or</u> you have a wetting accident.

Date	Put 'T' for emptying your bladder in the toilet, 'W' if you were just wet	Time of Day	Did you need to empty your bladder urgently? Put 'N' for the Not Urgent, 'U' for Urgent, 'E' for Extremely Urgent	Complete if you used the toilet after trying to 'Hold on'	
				How long did you hold on before starting?	Tick if you had an 'accident' while holding on

Fig. 17 'Holding' record chart

school. It may be continued at home in the evenings and at weekends. Although straightforward, most children will need a great deal of parental supervision in undertaking holding practice. The second approach described also requires an ability on the part of the child to recognize his first urge to urinate and to remember the holding routine. Whichever approach is used, a record should be kept to include: times of visits to the toilet, time for which the child 'held on', whether urgency was great, moderate or slight, daytime wetting incidents, and any accidents while trying to hold. Such records will show when a 'natural limit' is reached, and will indicate whether holding practice is being effective enough to be continued. A 'holding record chart' is illustrated in Fig. 17. It is useful for the columns recording visits to the toilet, urgency and daytime wettings to be completed for a one-week baseline period before starting holding practice, so that later progress can be measured against the position at the start.

Controlling urgency

Where a child experiences a definite and severe increase in urgency to urinate as he approaches the toilet, perhaps wetting before reaching it, it is useful to practice controlling this 'approach urgency'. Apart from reducing wetting problems on the way to the toilet, a reduction in sensitivity to this form of urgency can improve overall holding ability if successful.

Control of approach urgency can be helped by practicing holding for increasing periods just before starting the stream of urine into the toilet. The first step is for the child to get ready to urinate into the toilet as usual, but to try to count up to ten seconds before actually 'letting go' and starting the stream. A watch with a second hand is a useful aid, but most children can learn to count the seconds (although there is a tendency to rush the counting!). On reaching ten, urination is started. To hold on at this stage can be extremely difficult to a child with urgency, but if it can be achieved with practice, as it usually can, it represents the significant step forward of controlling urgency at its greatest level. Progress should as usual be recorded, on a sheet on which the number of seconds of successful 'holding off' can be written at each visit to the toilet (Fig. 18). It is often possible for this stage of control training to be practiced at school as well as at home.

When the child is consistently able to count to ten at or on the toilet, the second stage is to practice counting to ten at the toilet or bathroom

DAYTIME PANTS WETTING

Name .... Date Record Commences ....

FILL IN THE DATE EACH MORNING, AND FILL IN A NEW LINE EACH TIME YOU EMPTY YOUR BLADDER

DATE	TIME OF DAY	DID YOU NEED TO EMPTY YOUR BLADDER URGENTLY? PUT 'N' FOR NOT URGENT, 'U' FOR URGENT, 'E' FOR EXTREMELY URGENT	HOW MANY 'STOPS' TO COUNT TO TEN DID YOU MAKE?	IF YOU DIDN'T REACH TEN AT THE TOILET, HOW FAR DID YOU COUNT?

Fig. 18 Record chart for use when 'counting' to reduce approach urgency

door as well. When this can be achieved consistently and confidently, a further one or two 'stops' to count to ten can be added to other convenient stages en route to the toilet. Effectively, this routine aims to weaken the hold of the approach to the toilet over urgency, by partially dismantling it. By starting at or on the toilet itself and then only moving to count at earlier stages in the visit to the toilet as progress is made, the child is nearest the toilet when his risk of an accident is greatest.

Pelvic floor exercises

Figure 2 illustrates the importance of the pelvic floor muscles in controlling the outflow from the bladder. The pelvic floor comprises a powerful wedge of muscles between the legs, through which the urethra and rectum, and in girls the vagina, pass to reach the outside. The organs of the abdomen, including the bladder, lie inside a basin whose sides are largely formed by the bones of the pelvis and whose base is formed by the pelvic floor muscles.

From the function of the pelvic floor muscles in starting, preventing and stopping urination, as described in Chapter 2, it will be realized that exercises aimed at improving the strength and control of the pelvic floor can be helpful in reducing problems such as urgency or stress incontinence.

Many mothers will be familiar with the pelvic floor exercises they were taught to use after childbirth in order to regain good bladder control. Most of these exercises can also be used by children suffering from urgency or stress incontinence, alone or linked with daytime wetting.

Two useful pelvic floor exercises for children involve practice in raising the pelvic floor and holding it 'up' for brief periods. In the first, the child should stand with legs slightly apart, or lie on his back with knees bent, and practice pulling the pelvic floor up into his body towards the inside of the abdomen, holding it there for a short period, and then letting it relax again. When proficient at this, he can practice pulling it in and up in steps, rather like a lift, pausing at each stage. He may start with two stages, and then see how many separate 'floors' he can make the 'lift' stop at. Pulling the pelvic floor up is like 'tightening up' as if to prevent diarrhoea; the child may usefully place his hand on the pelvic floor to feel whether the movement inwards and upwards is taking place. He should not cheat by simply contracting the buttocks. This exercise should be repeated at least twice a day for five minute periods.

The second exercise is to practice using the pelvic floor actually to control the stream of urine when empying the bladder. The child should start the stream off and then practice stopping and restarting it, at least once on each visit, by pulling the pelvic floor up by its own contraction and then letting it fall again.

In either of these exercises, the usefulness of continuing to practice should be assessed according to progress recorded on a chart giving a rating of urgency at each urination (as is included in the holding chart in Fig. 17), together with a record of actual pants wettings.

Coping with smell

It is an unpleasant but familiar fact that an unpleasant smell is associated with wetting, particularly when clothing is wet by day. This often causes rejection and teasing by other children. Apart from regular and thorough washing, there is one very helpful measure that can be taken to reduce the problem of smell. This is to dust the clothing and affected skin liberally with a powder sold by chemists under the name of 'Mycil'. Sold primarily as a treatment for athlete's foot, this preparation acts against the bacteria that are responsible for much of the stale urine smell, which can be quite markedly reduced as a result.

Formal treatments

Apart from measures already described, the professional treatment of daytime urinary control problems by doctors and others centres upon the treatment of any infection present, the use of medicines, or, less commonly, on the use of a daytime equivalent to the night-time enuresis alarm or 'buzzer'. It is worth noting again here that it is quite common for daytime problems to improve to some extent if a night-time alarm is used with success to treat the bedwetting that is usually associated with daytime pants wetting.

In a very few cases, the doctor may diagnose some other physical problem lying behind the bladder control problem, and prescribe a suitable treatment or suggest further investigations.

Treatment of infection

The parents of a daytime wetter or a child with severe urgency or frequency should consult their doctor to check whether an infection is present. If so, it might be the cause of the difficulty, or at least it may aggravate it, keep it in existence, and defeat attempts to reduce it. Treatment of infection, usually by medication selected following analysis of a urine sample, may remove bladder control problems, but one should be prepared to use other approaches as well in case it does not. Even where an infection reduces control, removal of the infection does not always restore full control again.

Medicines

The medicines that a doctor may prescribe to treat daytime wetting are the same as those likely to be used in treating night wetting. Common drugs used are Tofranil, Tryptizol, Tyrimide and Cetiprin, but there is a range of others and it is therefore useful to record progress to report back to the doctor for a change of drug if necessary. Different drugs seem to suit different children. As in drug treatment of bedwetting, the aim is to reduce the responsiveness of the bladder to its contents of urine, and thus increase functional capacity and holding ability. All drug treatments for problems of bladder control seem to share a tendency towards relapse to wetting when the drug is stopped, whether it is stopped suddenly or gradually, and it is therefore helpful to try one or more of the self-help procedures already described as well. For some children, however, medication alone does do the trick permanently.

Daytime enuresis alarm or 'buzzer'

An enuresis alarm for use with daytime pants wetting can be obtained, but is a rare form of treatment because of the difficulty of using it outside the privacy of the home. It works on the same principle as the more common alarm or buzzer for bedwetting at night. Daytime alarms are designed to be worn in the clothing, and therefore are usually far smaller than the often bulky bedwetting alarm box, being suitable for wearing in a pocket, attached to the waistband, or slipped into a specially sewn-in pouch. The urine detector usually takes the form of electrode wires contained inside a soft cloth strip worn in the crotch or front of the pants, positioned and held in place by a sewn pouch or tapes where it will become wet as soon as urination begins. This type of apparatus is illustrated in Fig. 19.

Much of what has already been said about the night-time enuresis alarm in Chapters 4 and 5 applies to the daytime buzzer also. The alarm sound is triggered as soon as the detector pad in the pants becomes wet on accidental urination, and the sudden sound produces muscle contraction (including contraction of the pelvic floor) that tends to turn off the urine stream until the toilet can be reached. This holding reaction eventually becomes linked to bladder fullness. On hearing the sound, the child should try to hold on and make for the toilet to finish off. The alarm should be switched off as is convenient, and then reset afterwards ready for the next time. A clean and dry detector pad will be needed; the wet one being washed through and left to dry (possibly in the airing cupboard). Two or three detector pads will be required. As in treating bedwetting a record chart should be kept to monitor progress; day

DAYTIME PANTS WETTING

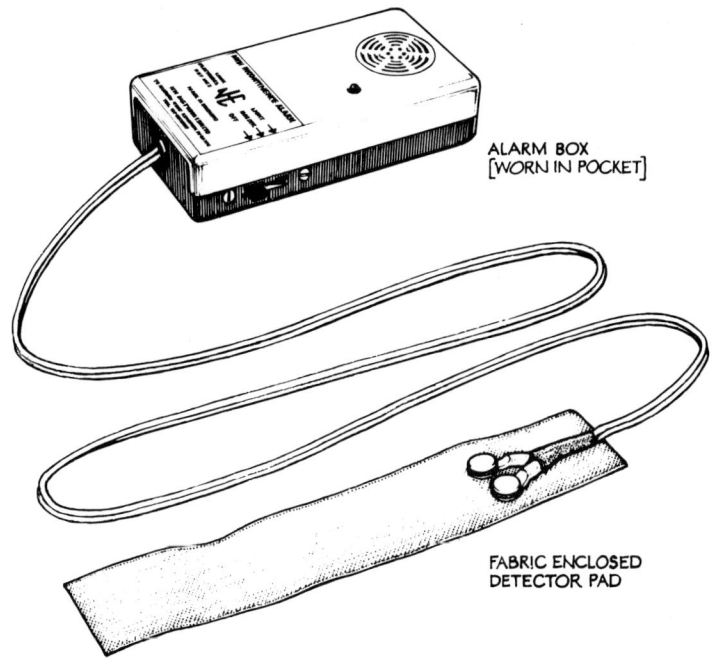

Fig. 19 The daytime 'buzzer'

wetting incidents can be recorded on a chart such as that in Fig. 10. Again, use of a day time alarm may be supported by the self-help procedures already described to assist the development of holding ability and reduction of urgency.

Although daytime alarm treatment is really only usable in private at home, loud alarm sounds on wetting not being practical at school or elsewhere, it is worth considering if more common and straightforward treatments have not succeeded. The alarm may then be worn while the child is in the house, for a reasonable period each day. It is helpful to start early in the school holidays at a time of year when the child is most likely to be playing or otherwise occupied indoors.

Teaching daytime control to the mentally handicapped

Problems of incontinence are common with children who have a mental handicap, and it is often possible to improve daytime bladder control, sometimes quite markedly, by a carefully structured training programme.

The essence of such a training programme is firstly to analyse as precisely and objectively as possible the ways in which your child falls short of adequate bladder control, secondly to plan a training programme to build up the necessary skills – in small, steadily progressive steps – and thirdly to record progress over a training period (which may be a matter of months), adapting the training programme according to its recorded results.

Analysing the problem

The basis of analysing a child's difficulties in the field of daytime bladder control is consideration and observation of his performance in each of the fundamental skills described in Chapter 2. A concise and accurate description of what he does do can lead to a definition of what he needs to learn to do, and of the paths he needs help to take. In describing what he does, and later recording any changes, it is useful to note in a special diary exactly what a video-camera would see him doing – to produce a 'script' of his actions that would be sufficient for an actor to repeat the important elements of his toilet behaviour. It is particularly important to note events and actions in their proper sequence, and to look for common basic patterns.

An important point to bear in mind in analysing the problem is the need to allow for the possible effects of any physical handicap. It is also important to remember that while in many handicapped children bladder control can be improved by careful training, this is not so in every case, the improvement does not necessarily reach full normal control, and much consistent, hard and painstaking work is involved.

Planning and using a training programme

Once you have identified one or more toileting skills that need developing, a training programme may be planned following straightforward learning principles. Much trial and error must be expected in finding the right combination of principles for a particular child, and to overcome the practical problems and the unexpected setbacks that often occur. Continued observation and noting of the child's actions while toileting provides the information to guide the development of the right training programme.

Rewarding desired actions is a simple but often surprisingly powerful form of training. Praise, a hug, a sweet even, can be used as an effective reward to strengthen and increase the probability of an action. The important points to follow in using a reward programme are:

1. Reward small, easily and specifically defined 'bits' of behaviour.
2. Be quite clear as to what the child must do to achieve his reward, and avoid the temptation to reward 'a good try' or, worse, giving a reward to 'make up' for a failure.
3. Give the reward immediately it has been earned.
4. If using sweets or food (bits of flavoured breakfast cereal are often very popular), praise the child as well. If you praise just *before* giving the food reward, the effect of your praise will actually be strengthened by its association with the food.
5. Small rewards for small achievements are more effective than waiting for a big reward for a major achievement.
6. Record your child's progress — if there is no more progress, try a different reward; if that does not work, try breaking the action wanted into even smaller steps to be rewarded; if that fails, rethink the strategy.
7. Do not be afraid to guide the child in the actions to perform, rewarding him however much guidance was needed — the guidance can be faded out later as he 'picks up' on his own.
8. Once an action is well-established, begin missing out the occasional reward, then phasing the rewards out from 'every time' to 'very infrequent'. Every-time rewarding is strongest for training; occasional and reducing rewarding helps to stabilize what has been learned as a relatively permanent action.

Three basic reward programmes are given below, with examples of how they might work out in practice.

1 *Simple rewarding.* When a necessary piece of toileting behaviour does occur sometimes, but not often enough, its frequency can be increased in many cases simply by rewarding it whenever it does occur. The rewards can be explained to a child who can understand. (It is also worth noting that the same strategy can be useful with non-handicapped children.)

An example of simple reward training is its use with a child who only very occasionally uses the toilet to urinate or defaecate, more often wetting or soiling his underclothing. Every time the child urinates or defaecates in the toilet, he is given praise, a hug and a sweet he likes immediately he has 'performed'. His parents will record the number of toiletings each day to see whether the number is increasing, or whether the strategy needs rethinking. They will prompt and guide the child where it helps, phasing this out as he 'picks up'. Once the daily frequency of successful toiletings rather than 'accidents' has reliably increased and guidance is phased out, the sweet will be left out once every three toiletings, then more often until it is rarely given and finally dropped. The special praise and hug can then be reduced until toileting is 'kept going' by the occasional congratulations and hug only. (Contrary to the common expectation, use of sweets or other rewards can usually be phased out or replaced by praise alone — it is far rarer than one might think that a child will learn to 'do it, but only for sweets'.)

2 *'Shaping'*. Often the piece of behaviour one wants the child to use in order to improve his continence never occurs, and therefore is just not there to be rewarded. 'Shaping' is a reward technique useful in such cases. The object is to mould or 'shape' the action wanted by rewarding the child (again, by praise or perhaps a small piece of something he likes to eat) for every move in the right direction. The principle is the same as the party game in which a person is guided towards some object or action by being told he is 'hot' or 'cold'.

As an example, a child who simply never sits on the toilet, and indeed may be rather afraid of it, can often be shaped into sitting on it when told to. At the beginning, he may be told to 'go to toilet' (or whatever the usual family words are), and as soon as he makes the slightest move in the right direction, rewarded. When he moves each time, he must advance further before his reward, and so on until he must actually sit on the toilet to receive it. With one autistic boy, the author gave raisins as rewards, first when the boy left his chair, then (standing ahead of him) half-way to the door of the room, at the door, on the landing, at the bathroom door, in the bathroom, standing by the pot, touching the pot, and finally only when he had sat on the pot. Verbal instruction, gentle physical guidance, and example can be used to encourage and 'lead' the next step; the rewards effectively fuel the performance of the sequence. Once it is established, the rewards for a complete shaped action can be phased out in the usual way.

3 *'Chaining'*. Shaping is one way of building actions up into a complex piece of behaviour that does not occur on its own. 'Chaining' is a technique in which a sequence of quite separate actions can be linked

together to form a complex piece of behaviour. To build a 'chain' of actions (such as removing clothing, sitting on the toilet, cleaning up, replacing clothing, flushing, and washing hands), the first step can be taught and rewarded, then instead of phasing out the reward, the next is added so that both must be performed before the reward and so on. The secret is not to try to achieve the whole chain of events in one go, but to add the next link in the chain only when the previous ones are well-established and well linked together — always rewarding when the latest link to be added is achieved. The parent will do for the child all the stages following this. When the last in the desired chain of events has been added, the reward for the whole sequence can be phased out gradually in the usual manner.

One can build up a chain of events by teaching and rewarding the first action first, but it is often more useful and convenient to teach the *last* link first and then build the chain backwards. An example will clarify these techniques: the sequence of actions forming the desired chain might be those in replacing underpants and trousers after using the toilet. The links in the chain would be: stand up, hold underpants, pull underpants up, position them properly, let go, hold trousers, pull trousers up, position properly, do up zip, tuck in, do up belt. (Different children may need the sequence broken down into more or fewer steps.) To build the chain *forwards*, the child is first shown how to hold his pants, rewarded when he achieves this, and then shown how to pull them up, and rewarded when he has done both in the right order — and so on until he achieves the whole sequence to receive his reward after doing his belt up. Until he reaches this point, his parent will take over after he has done his part of the chain. To build the chain *backwards*, the parent will begin by doing each stage for him up to fastening his belt, teaching him to do this last bit to finish off, and rewarding him for doing it. When he can do this, the next stage is added to 'his' part of the chain so that he takes over to tuck in and fasten his belt to gain his reward — and so on until he can do the whole sequence without a parent starting him off. The reward is always at the end of the chain, and is not phased out until the whole chain is carried out reliably.

The previous paragraphs have outlined some of the basic programmes that can be used in daytime toilet training of mentally handicapped children. The principles used are simple and fairly obvious; the skill and effort lies in focusing straightforward training principles such as in-structing and rewarding the child for small steps in the right direction, into a systematic training programme with the right strategy for the particular child involved, and with a record of progress to indicate the success or need for change in a programme. The principles are few and simple, rather like the rules of chess, but as in chess, the combination of those rules into a successful strategy can be both challenging and difficult. There are pitfalls — it is all too easy, for instance, to find that a carefully built 'chain' becomes useless because a 'wrong' link (such as the child wetting on the way to an otherwise perfect use of the toilet) accidentally appears and is rewarded at the end of the chain before one realizes what is happening.

The purpose of mentioning such pitfalls is not to discourage parents from trying to design and carry out their own training programme, but to stress the patience and effort needed, to point out that training can often need major redesigning at various points, and that one must expect some disappointments before achieving eventual success. The effectiveness of programmes such as those described can be increased by many parents if they are able to secure the advice of someone experienced in planning and carrying out this form of training. It is well worth consulting one's 'contacts' amongst special school staff and educational or clinical (hospital) psychologists to see if such a person is locally available.

7

Soiling

Soiling one's underclothing with faeces ('encopresis') is one of the most humiliating problems a child could have. It is a problem that is more common amongst children with a day or night wetting problem than amongst non-wetting children, it is more common in boys than girls, and it is more common where there is a mental handicap. It is also a problem where there are relevant physical handicaps. Children and parents may be reassured that although soiling is more common in bedwetting or day wetting children than in others, the boy or girl who has bowel control but not full bladder control will not start to soil just because he has other incontinence problems.

Soiling is usually a daytime problem; soiling at night is very rare and needs investigation by a doctor. A medical opinion should however be sought for all children basically unable to control the bowel. As with wetting, a physical cause is rare but needs checking.

It is common for children with a soiling problem to be 'difficult' in varying ways, since soiling results in such a social problem for the child concerned, and is so damaging to his self-esteem. Many become blasé about their problem – having little option but to develop a tough skin about it. Most have desperate strategies to try to avoid discovery when they have soiled, often hiding their soiled clothing. It is important to agree with a soiling child, at the outset, an acceptable means of coping with soiled clothing, such as a covered bucket of water containing disinfectant or nappy-sanitizer.

Types of soiling

Retention-with-overflow

This is the most common form of soiling. It will be remembered from Chapter 2 (and Fig. 3) that the rectum, as the final section of the bowel, is

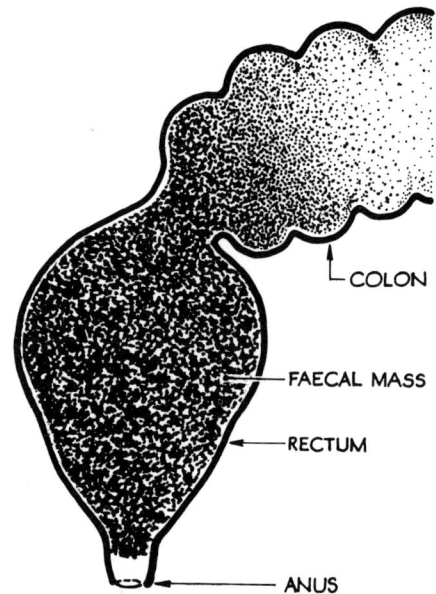

Fig. 20 The rectum loaded with a faecal mass

normally an empty tube which gives rise to the sensation of needing to defaecate when faeces enter it and stretch its walls (see Fig. 20). In normal bowel control, faeces enter and stretch the rectum on a more or less regular cycle, leading to defaecation in the toilet.

A soiling problem can arise when the urgency signal arising from the rectum being stretched by faeces breaks down. This happens if faeces are held in the rectum instead of being emptied, leaving it stretched for too long. This leads to the rectum becoming adjusted to being stretched, and the stretching therefore ceasing to give rise to the normal feelings of urgency to defaecate. The child, no longer feeling urgency to empty his bowel, still needs to do so however. If the bowel continues to remain unemptied, new waste material arriving in the rectum from above stretches the rectum even further and builds up a growing blockage of faeces. The size of this mass can make attempts at emptying difficult and even painful — and eventually the mass of waste matter back along the large intestine can be felt from the outside, rising on the front left side of the child's abdomen. Soiling itself begins when mainly liquid waste matter, having to go somewhere, finds its way out around the solid mass of faeces. The walls of the rectum and the circles of muscle which usually control any escape of faeces, being over-stretched, cannot then control the inevitable leakage of liquid matter into the clothing – usually without the over-stretched lower bowel informing the child that leakage is happening.

A retention-with-overflow problem can start when a child for some reason fails over a prolonged period to empty his bowel in response to feelings of urgency 'to go'. The danger signal that problems are starting is often the loss of the feeling of urgency – either by letting it pass away once felt without using the toilet (leaving the rectum stretched), or through feelings of urgency becoming weak and infrequent. Reasons for a child not emptying his bowel despite feeling the urge to do so can be quite minor and easily overlooked. Some children tend to ignore the urge when they are engrossed in some activity, and many avoid using school toilets. It is remarkable how many school toilets have no lockable doors or no paper, and it is worth noting that the toilets are usually the least supervised areas of the school, and are often the scene of teasing and bullying, or are occupied by those engaged in illicit activities such as smoking. Children may avoid defaccation if it is painful, as it can be if there is a small fissure or split of the anus, or if the child is simply constipated. Some younger children are simply afraid of toilets – particularly strange ones.

Apart from those children whose soiling problem represents a loss of previous control, there are some who never developed a regular cycle of rectal filling followed by toileting, with the resultant risk of retention with overflow.

Non-control

Some children with a soiling problem do not have any retention problem, but simply do not, or have not learned, to use the toilet for defaecation. The bowel is emptied when the sensation of urgency arises, but in places other than the toilet. This can happen where there is a mental handicap and with a very few otherwise normal children; particularly the young child who has not yet succeeded in limiting his defaecations to the toilet or pot alone. Thus the problem is really a persistence to a rather late age (say, three-plus) of the accidents away from the toilet that happen in the early stages of acquiring bowel control.

It is rare, but must be stressed, that a child can have a physical problem which renders him unable to control the emptying of his bowel, without having any retention problem. This needs to be diagnosed through medical investigation.

Staining

The *amount* of faeces in the underclothing is important in assessing a soiling problem. Very many children (and adults) stain their underclothing with 'skid marks' quite normally, and this does not indicate anything of concern. In some cases, a child's soiling may be no more than particularly heavy staining of this type, resulting from inefficient wiping after perfectly normal defaecation.

Countermeasures to soiling

Medical examination is required in cases of severe or persistent soiling, mainly to determine whether there is a retained mass of faeces in the rectum. If so, an enema may be required to clear the retained mass. Subsequent treatment of soiling is relatively logical and straightforward, but requires persistence and meticulous routine over a period of time. The simplest retention with overflow cases can sometimes clear up relatively quickly, however, if the right routine is selected and strictly followed. Apart from laxatives, the concentration in treatment is more upon toileting routine than upon drugs.

As with all treatments and management procedures described in this book, a record of progress is an important aid in confirming the usefulness of, or alternatively the need to change, the strategy being used. A simple record chart suitable for the purpose is illustrated in Fig. 21.

Regular toileting

Many children with a soiling problem simply do not use the toilet regularly for defaecation. The first step in trying to solve a soiling problem is to ensure that the child does visit the toilet and try to empty his bowel there at a regular time at least once a day. Cleanliness cannot be expected without reasonably frequent use of the toilet, and a regular cycle of rectal filling and defaecation is an important element in normal control. Some cases of soiling can be resolved, surprisingly perhaps, by doing nothing more complicated that ensuring regular toileting.

Please fill this record in every evening at bed-time. Put 'S' if the child had soiled his or her underclothes with faeces at any time during the day. Put 'C' if the child was clean throughout the day.

Name _____   Record commencing _____

	Week 1	Week 2	Week 3	Week 4	Week 5	Week 6	Week 7	Week 8	Week 9	Week 10	Week 11	Week 12
Monday												
Tuesday												
Wednesday												
Thursday												
Friday												
Saturday												
Sunday												

Fig. 21 Record chart for soiling problems

Intensive toileting*

Where a child has developed a severe retention-with-overflow problem, and may have lost the urgency signal through continuous stretching of the rectum, a more intensive toileting routine will probably be needed. Medical opinion should however be sought first, as the initial step may well need to be removal of the retained faeces from the rectum by an enema.

The object, once any serious retention is removed, is to keep the rectum empty — to avoid any further build-up of retained faeces, and to allow the walls of the rectum to regain their sensitivity to being stretched by the arrival of new faeces. Intensive toileting is simple, but *must* be carried out strictly and consistently. It involves three elements:

1. A mild laxative (such as Senokot) taken last thing at night (checking with your doctor first that there is no reason against this for your particular case). The laxative will make the child more likely to defaecate in the morning, and will ensure that the faeces are soft and easy to evacuate, not likely to start 'setting' again into a retained mass.
2. A warm drink after breakfast every morning. It is its warmth, rather than what drink it is, that matters. The warm drink serves to set in motion the waves of muscular contractions ('persistalsis') along the tubes of the gut, that help to push the faeces out from the rectum.
3. Twenty minutes after the warm drink, the child should visit the toilet and try to empty his bowel. This is generally the time taken for the muscular contractions triggered by the drink to reach the rectum. With both the laxative and the warm drink, the child will be visiting the toilet at the time defaecation is most likely.

This intensive toileting routine should be maintained until soiling has stopped and has stayed away for at least two weeks. One should allow up to three months for this, although in some cases a quite rapid response can occur. The treatment is successful in a significant proportion, but certainly not all, cases of retention-with-overflow soiling in children. Although the research is limited, the chances of success in a given case are probably in the region of fifty/fifty.

Once two weeks free of soiling have been achieved, the laxative may be discontinued, but the regular toileting pattern should be continued

* This treatment technique was developed by my former colleague, Dr. Gordon Young.

permanently, and it is helpful if the warm drink is continued as well.

If the progress record shows little improvement after a few weeks, the warm drink, 20 minute wait and toileting, can be repeated after each meal as well as after breakfast.

Many parents are surprised at first when laxatives are suggested for soiling children, although the reader can appreciate their value because of the retention problem. It is important however to stress that soiling with liquid faeces where a child has retention-with-overflow has nothing at all to do with diarrhoea, and anti-diarrhoea mixtures should *not* be used. They will simply aggravate the problem by adding to the retained mass.

In this section, laxatives such as Senokot have been discussed, but some doctors may prescribe suppositories for the same purpose to achieve a rather greater and more direct effect.

Reacting to urgency

From Chapter 2 it will be recalled that although the bladder is normally partially full, the rectum should normally be kept empty. To prevent the build up of a retained mass and resultant loss of the vital stretch-urgency signal from the rectum when faeces enter it, a child who feels urgency to defaecate should always respond to it by visiting the toilet as soon as possible. By doing this, he will avoid leaving the rectum stretched and full for more than short periods, thus ensuring that he will continue to receive the urgency signal when faeces pass into the rectum and need emptying. Regular or intensive toilet training will encourage this to happen and at roughly the same time or times each day.

The golden rule for the child is: *when you have the urge to empty your bowel, use the toilet before the urge has time to pass away*. If the child does let the urge pass away, he should still defaecate as soon as possible – the urge does not disappear because he no longer needs to go, but because his rectum is becoming dangerously used to being stretched. The faeces are still there to be emptied.

Diet

It is worth reviewing the diet of a child with a soiling problem. A poor diet is unlikely to cause severe soiling, but it can adversely affect bowel regularity and the consistency of the faeces enough to put what bowel control there is under severe strain, and to inhibit progress in relieving soiling.

A diet tending to lead to 'loose' faeces can cause problems where regular toileting is not established and there is a degree of 'non-control'. One leading towards constipation can make defaecation difficult and encourage retention. The aim is a reasonably balanced diet with a good proportion of 'roughage'.

Reward training

In 'non-control' cases, particularly with the mentally handicapped, the reward-training principle described in the last chapter can be used to train the child to use the toilet as is necessary to stay clean. With a non-control problem, in normal as well as mentally handicapped children, it is helpful to give rewards for two things. Firstly, for producing faeces in the toilet, and secondly for periods of keeping the pants clean (the child can be 'checked' at intervals).

The use of rewards is helpful with many children having poor bowel control, but needs adapting according to the particular child. The handicapped child or the young child can be checked and closely supervised, and can be rewarded immediately — either with (perhaps) something edible, or with the award of points to be saved up (rather like cash) towards something larger. With an older child, points or even coins may be used, or the child may be trusted to keep his own records and points system. A simple record, without back-up rewards as such, can sometimes have the same effect as a basic reward system.

Accepting the toilet

An important factor in the relief of soiling for many children is encouragement to use the toilet when necessary away from home, particularly at school. The problem of school toilets without privacy or paper has already been mentioned; these can put a child off toileting at school sufficiently to cause bowel problems. It is easy to be put off by 'adverse toilets', as many adults will realize if they have ever encountered abroad the type of toilet which requires one to straddle a hole in the floor.

Children can be helped to use school toilets by very simple strategies, depending upon their particular worry. A pad of toilet paper can be carried from home, an arrangement can be reached with the teacher for the child to visit the toilet during class, when other children are not there, or a trusted friend may 'stand guard' outside the door. The soiling problem at school of one patient of the author's was resolved when he was equipped with a steel rule to hold the school toilet door closed.

A very small number of children are actually afraid of sitting on the toilet. The most useful solution to this problem is to take the child towards the toilet, and eventually to sit on it, *gradually*, in small steps. One should start at a distance at which the child is happy, and simply 'introduce' him a little closer (and for a little longer) each attempt. Praise and specific reward can help in addition.

Glossary

Terms used in this book, and which may be helpful in discussions with the family doctor or a specialist.

ALARM: The enuresis alarm, 'buzzer' or 'bell-and-pad'. A device to treat bedwetting which produces a loud sound when detector mats in the bed become wet.
ANUS: The outlet of the bowel, through which the body's waste matter (faeces) passes to the outside.
APPROACH URGENCY: A tendency for the need to empty the bladder to become greater as one approaches the toilet.
BASELINE: A record of toiletings, or of bladder or bowel control problems, kept before beginning any form of treatment to measure the extent of a problem, help in choosing goals for treatment, and for comparison with later records to measure progress.
BELL-AND-PAD: One name for the enuresis alarm. (The very earliest alarms used bells rather than buzzer sounds.)
BLADDER: The muscular sac which stores the body's urine until it can be emptied to the outside.
BUZZER: Another name for the enuresis alarm.
CATHETER: Small tube inserted through the urethra into the bladder, usually as a means of emptying it artificially of urine, or in testing the way it is functioning.
CETIPRIN: A drug used in treating wetting problems.
CHAINING: The use of reward learning techniques to build up complex toileting behaviours (particularly with the mentally handicapped), by linking together a series (or 'chain') of small steps.
CHART: A progress record of toileting, wetting or soiling.
CLASSICAL CONDITIONING: Learning through the association of one thing with another.
CLOSURE MECHANISM: The system which shuts off the outlet of the bladder, involving the pelvic floor muscles.
COLON: The lower part of the bowel, leading to the final section or rectum.
CONDITIONING: A basic form of learning actions or reactions,

through association or the influence of their consequences.
DEFAECATION: The action of emptying faeces from the body.
DETECTOR MAT: A special wire mesh, metal foil or plastic-and-metal mat or pair of mats, placed in the bed to detect bedwetting and trigger the alarm sound in enuresis alarm treatment.
DETRUSOR: The thin muscle that forms the walls of the bladder.
DISCRIMINATIVE STIMULUS: A signal recognized by the body as predicting whether the consequences of a particular action will be pleasant or unpleasant – rather like a 'traffic light' signalling whether or not to go ahead.
DIURNAL ENURESIS: Daytime pants-wetting.
ELECTRODES: The two metal parts of the detector mats used with an enuresis alarm.
ENCOPRESIS: Soiling the clothing with faeces.
ENEMA: Substance inserted through the anus to empty the rectum of faeces artificially.
ENURESIS: Bedwetting or daytime wetting.
ENURESIS ALARM: See ALARM.
FAECES: The body's solid waste matter, passed from the bowel through the anus to the outside.
FALSE ALARM: The triggering of an enuresis alarm at night when the child has not wet the bed – usually because of sweat.
FAMILY HISTORY: Wetting and soiling problems in members of the family other than the patient – these problems tending to run in families.
FLUID RESTRICTION: Reducing the amount a child drinks, or stopping him drinking in the evening.
FUNCTIONAL BLADDER CAPACITY: The amount of urine the bladder has become used to holding before signalling the need to be emptied.
GIGGLE MICTURITION: A form of daytime wetting, so called because it is often triggered by laughing, in which the bladder empties completely once a 'leak' is started by some bodily strain on the bladder (such as in laughing, coughing or sneezing).
HOLDING: Keeping urine in the bladder for a period; trying to increase the amount of urine the bladder can hold before needing to be emptied (the functional bladder capacity) by postponing urination for brief periods after urgency is felt.
INCONTINENCE: Passing urine or faeces involuntarily.
INDIVIDUAL DIFFERENCES: The often quite great differences in

bladder and bowel control between children that are quite normal and are simply some of the many differences between one person and another.

KIDNEYS: The two organs that filter liquid waste materials from the blood and produce urine.

LIFTING: Waking a child or taking him from his bed at night to use the toilet.

MICTURITION: Technical term for passing urine.

MSU: Mid-stream specimen of urine – a urine sample for laboratory testing to discover infection or other indications of abnormality, made up of the later rather than first part of the stream of urine passed.

MYCIL: Powder, sold for the treatment of athlete's foot, which also reduces the smell of urine on the skin.

NOCTURNAL ENURESIS: Bedwetting.

OPERANT CONDITIONING: Learning in which an action is strengthened or weakened in the future by the pleasantness or unpleasantness of its consequences.

OVERLEARNING: Increased drinking at the end of alarm treatment of bedwetting, to strengthen the control learned through treatment and reduce the likelihood of a relapse.

PELVIC FLOOR: The sheet of internal muscles between the legs which support the bladder and whose relaxation and contraction play an important part in controlling the bladder.

PERISTALSIS: The waves of muscle contraction that run along the gut to squeeze its contents along.

PLACEBO EFFECT: The tendency of all treatments to have some good effect, whatever they are, and without any obvious explanation.

PLAY THERAPY: Treatment in which a therapist tries to help a child through play.

PRIMARY ENURESIS: Wetting that has lasted ever since infancy.

PSYCHOTHERAPY: Treatment which (usually) involves looking for meanings behind a child's actions and problems – often through talking or play.

POTTING: Toilet training technique of placing the child on the pot and encouraging urination or defaecation.

RECTUM: The end section of the bowel.

REINFORCEMENT: Strengthening a needed action for the future by praising or rewarding the child when it happens.

RELAPSE: The recurrence of a problem after it has been successfully treated.

GLOSSARY

RETENTION WITH OVERFLOW: (of faeces); when liquid faeces seep around a mass of solid faeces that has built up in the rectum, to soil the underclothes (sometimes mistaken for diarrhoea). (Of urine); when urine cannot be passed normally to empty the bladder completely, the bladder can overfill and result in leakage of urine.
REWARDING: Use of rewards to strengthen or reinforce a desirable action.
SECONDARY ENURESIS: Wetting that has begun after the child has been reliably dry for some time.
SENOKOT: A common laxative — sometimes used to prevent retention with overflow of faeces.
SHAPING: Method of building up a needed complex action by rewarding any of the child's actions which take him closer to the desired behaviour. Useful in teaching toileting skills to the mentally handicapped.
SOILING: Passing faeces into the pants.
STAINING: Slight soiling of the underpants with faeces.
STAGGERED WAKING: Lifting a child to use the pot or toilet at different times each night.
STAR CHART: A record chart of wetting or soiling on which the child is rewarded by putting stars for 'dry' or 'clean' days or nights as appropriate.
STRESS INCONTINENCE: The 'leakage' of urine from the body when the bladder is under pressure through an action such as laughing, coughing or sneezing.
STRETCH REFLEX: The reaction of the rectum to being stretched open by the presence of faeces — a sensation of urgency to defaecate and contraction to expel faeces during defaecation.
SUPPOSITORY: Inserted through the anus into the rectum to assist defaecation.
TOFRANIL: Drug used in treating wetting problems.
TOILET DREAM: Where the child dreams he is at the toilet when wetting the bed.
TRYPTIZOL: Drug used in treating wetting problems.
TYRIMIDE: Drug used in treating wetting problems.
URETER: The tube which takes urine from each kidney to the bladder.
URETHRA: The tube from the bladder to the outside of the body, through which urine is passed on urination.
URINE: The liquid waste of the body, stored in the bladder and emptied through the urethra.
URINATION: Emptying the bladder of urine.

Further Reading

Azrin, N., Foxx, R. *Toilet Training in Less than a Day*. London: Macmillan, 1975. (An intensive toilet training programme.)

Kolvin, I., MacKeith, R. C., Meadow, R. S. (eds.) *Bladder Control and Enuresis*. London: Heinemann Medical, 1973. (Collected research reports and major reviews on many aspects of enuresis.)

Mandelstam, Dorothy. *Incontinence*. London: Heinemann Medical, 1977 (through The Disabled Living Foundation). (A valuable handbook for problems of incontinence in adults.)

Montgomery, Eileen. *Regaining Bladder Control*. Bristol: Wright, 1974. (Contains useful pelvic floor exercises.)